The Political Economy of Health and Healthcare

The healthcare sector is one of the fastest growing areas of social and public spending worldwide, and it is expected to increase its government shares of GDP in the near future. Truly global in its scope, this book presents a unified, structured understanding of how the design of a country's health institutions influence its healthcare activities and outcomes. Building on the 'public choice' tradition in political economy, the authors explore how patient-citizens interact with their country's political institutions to determine the organisation of the health system. The book discusses a number of institutional influences of a health system, such as federalism, the nature of collective action, electoral competition, constitutional designs, political ideologies, the welfare effects of corruption and lobbying and, more generally, the dynamics of change. Whilst drawing on the theoretical concepts of political economy, this book describes an institution-grounded analysis of health systems in an accessible way. We hope it will appeal to both undergraduate and graduate students studying health economics, health policy and public policy. More generally, it can help health policy community to structure ideas about policy and institutional reform.

JOAN COSTA-FONT is an associate professor of the Department of Health Policy, at the London School of Economics and Political Science. He is a research fellow of IZA and CESIfo and has been Harkness Fellow at Harvard University and Visiting Fellow at Paris Dauphine University, UCL, Boston College, Oxford University, amongst other universities.

GILBERTO TURATI is a professor of Public Finance at the Department of Economics and Finance at the Università Cattolica del Sacro Cuore. He was Board Member of the European Public Choice Society (2012-2015) and is currently a Board Member of the Italian Society of Public Economics.

ALBERTO BATINTI is an associate professor of Economics at the International Business School Suzhou – Xi'an Jiaotong-Liverpool University and External Fellow at the Center for Health Economics at the University of Nottingham Ningbo China. He has published research papers in peer-reviewed academic journals as *Public Choice, The European Journal of Political Economy, Kyklos*, and *Health Economics.*

The Political Economy of Health and Healthcare

The Rise of the Patient Citizen

JOAN COSTA-FONT
London School of Economics and Political Science

GILBERTO TURATI
Università Cattolica del Sacro Cuore

ALBERTO BATINTI
Xi'an Jiaotong-Liverpool University

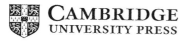

CAMBRIDGE
UNIVERSITY PRESS

CAMBRIDGE
UNIVERSITY PRESS

University Printing House, Cambridge CB2 8BS, United Kingdom

One Liberty Plaza, 20th Floor, New York, NY 10006, USA

477 Williamstown Road, Port Melbourne, VIC 3207, Australia

314–321, 3rd Floor, Plot 3, Splendor Forum, Jasola District Centre,
New Delhi – 110025, India

79 Anson Road, #06–04/06, Singapore 079906

Cambridge University Press is part of the University of Cambridge.

It furthers the University's mission by disseminating knowledge in the pursuit of
education, learning, and research at the highest international levels of excellence.

www.cambridge.org
Information on this title: www.cambridge.org/9781108474979
DOI: 10.1017/9781108653015

First published 2020

Printed in the United Kingdom by TJ International Ltd, Padstow Cornwall

A catalogue record for this publication is available from the British Library.

Library of Congress Cataloging-in-Publication Data
Names: Costa-Font, Joan, author. | Turati, Gilberto, 1971– author. | Batinti, Alberto,
    1978– author.
Title: The political economy of health and healthcare : the rise of the patient citizen /
    Joan Costa-Font, Gilberto Turati, Alberto Batinti.
Description: Cambridge ; New York, NY : Cambridge University Press, 2020. |
    Includes bibliographical references and index.
Identifiers: LCCN 2019045595 (print) | LCCN 2019045596 (ebook) |
    ISBN 9781108474979 (hardback) | ISBN 9781108468251 (paperback) |
    ISBN 9781108653015 (epub)
Subjects: LCSH: Medical policy. | Health systems agencies–Political aspects. | Health
    services administration–Political aspects. | Medical economics.
Classification: LCC RA393 .C682 2020 (print) | LCC RA393 (ebook) | DDC 362.1–dc23
LC record available at https://lccn.loc.gov/2019045595
LC ebook record available at https://lccn.loc.gov/2019045596

ISBN 978-1-108-47497-9 Hardback
ISBN 978-1-108-46825-1 Paperback

Contents

Figures

Tables

Preface

With the proliferation of academic journals and the increased importance attributed to research papers for academic careers, the tradition of writing book manuscripts has become less popular in social sciences. However, there still is a point in writing a book. Namely, to provide an 'unified overview' of a specific field of research. This is especially the case when the research produced in several disciplines, has set the foundations of an independent field of study which can be labelled as the 'political economy of health and healthcare'. Increasingly, scholars of different disciplines such as economics, politics, sociology and health sciences, among others, have produced a wealth of knowledge on how political institutions and processes influence the dynamics and performance of health systems. Most of these contributions, however, tend to be scattered, and often fail to communicate with each other when they probably should, for the discipline to continue advancing. The purpose of this book is to build a bridge between disciplines and help contribute to a unified perspective.

Our point of departure and cornerstone is that of designing a health system that attempts to improve the welfare of a 'patient citizen' (PC), which is the agent we focus our attention on. The PC is subject to at least two agency relationships which constrain its behaviour. First, as is typically acknowledged by health economists, citizens are (either current or potential) patients who engage in an agency relationship where a doctor acts as their advisor helping them navigate the health system and identify their healthcare demands. Second, in democratic states, with some statutory health insurance citizens have typically a constitutionally defined right to healthcare, pay mandatory taxes and other insurance contributions to help fund the health system. However, they also contribute with their votes to elect the representatives who will decide on their behalf with regards to health policy matters, including the organisation, financing and regulation of public and private health services. Government actions influence how much households pay for healthcare, whether they vaccinate their children at the right time and how many barriers they face in having access to healthcare services.

Although the health sector is one of the most dynamic areas of institutional reform, we still lack a 'unified' approach to examine health reforms that explicitly considers the role of political motivations in changing behaviour. To date, barely any book provides such a comprehensive overview of the role of political incentives in the functioning of health systems, that engages with wider and heterogeneous audiences. Although all the authors of this book are economists by training, we attempt to reach out beyond our discipline, and have done our best to avoid the use of equations and jargon. To that purpose, we have focused on describing general principles and empirical regularities rather than exploring in depth modelling and econometric applications. Intentionally, some of the evidence presented is descriptive, but we hope it can stimulate discussion on the matters examined, such as the role of democracies on health systems development, or the influence of a median voter, or whether a coalition of the 'ends against the middle' influences policy choices. It is worth mentioning that the book contains numerous citations for anyone interested in delving more deeply into each aspect discussed.

Much of the developments in the field of health economics has traditionally ignored the developments in political economy, and instead takes institutions as exogenous, and has centred around the principles of welfare economics or policy analysis. In contrast, here we are interested in the endogenous nature of policies and institutions, and we do not necessarily assume the existence of a planner, or a social welfare function. On the other hand, political science and sociological research in health does not attempt to engage with economists either, and the litertaure, to date tends to be very United States (US) centred. Finally, health research adopts a more pragmatic and empirical perspective, and often lacks the theoretical grounding that is typically developed by social science disciplines. This book can help to lay out some conceptual understanding of how to examine health reforms. For instance, we will attempt to identify under which circumstances lobbying benefits the patient citizen, and hence is welfare improving; or how different types of regulatory 'capture' lead to government failure; or the extent to which a country that engages with corruption will end up wasting important resources in the health system.

Inevitably, in writing a book with such a vast remit, we had to make some tough choices. First, we decided to employ rational choice institutionalism as a framework, that is, we ground most of our analysis with the public choice tradition of institutional study. However, we do not disregard the study of processes let alone the role of the historical evolution of institutions, nor the rules of the game in a society. When possible, we acknowledge that strategies and behaviours are context specific. Similarly, we explicitly consider explicitly the role of ideas and ideologies in framing health policy decisions. Second, we have mainly focused on those questions where there is already some research, often opting out of aspects that are not yet well researched or venturing to answer some questions tentatively. This has allowed us to identify areas for further research, which we plan to contribute ourselves in the future, and we encourage others to join us in the endeavour. Third, there have been important aspects such as the study of 'bureaucracies in healthcare' or the 'interactions of public and private healthcare' that could have deserved a full chapter, but this would have made the project 'never-ending'.

In deciding which matters to focus on, we have chosen what in our view are the most critical contributions in the field, and hence the book structure choosen is inevitably biased. However, this book is written to be a 'first edition', and we hope that soon we will write a new one that addresses some of the aspects on which we could not devote more space to this time around. In some circumstances we had the feeling of trying to hit a moving target, which just signals the great interest and attention that researchers in growing numbers around the world are paying to these topics.

The authors' order reflects their leading role in steering the book project, as well as historical additions to the project. While we consider this work a joint effort, Costa-Font took the lead on a first draft of Chapters 2, 3, 4 and 9, Turati on Chapters 1, 7 and 8, Batinti on Chapters 5, 6 and 10. All chapters have been co-written, and discussed at length.

This book could not have been possible without the encouragement of Roger Congleton, Adam Oliver, Alistair McGuire and the support of the Department of Health policy at the London School of Economics (LSE). We are very grateful to Jacob Lang for the enormous effort devoted to helping us with editing, putting it together and turning it into a coherent piece, as well as friends at the Cambridge University Press office, especially Phil Good and Tobias Ginsberg. We also thank three anonymous external reviewers for very valuable comments which helped us improve the book. We are indebted to the participants to the European Public Choice Society (EPCS) meeting in Cambridge, back in 2014, where we had the chance to discuss a number of matters around the political economy of health. To our knowledge, this was one of the very first dedicated sessions on the topic, and surely the place where the seed of this book was planted. Since then, almost every year, EPCS and American Public Choice Society (PCS) meetings have progressively included parallel sessions on health and healthcare. We see the interest in the political economy of health and healthcare as an upward trend as public health budgets are becoming increasing shares of government activities around the world, and not only in high income countries.

We hope you, the reader, enjoy the content of the book, which only attempts to make a first step towards the development of a fruitful area of interdisciplinary analysis of health policy and healthcare institutions. After all, all of us really are patient citizens looking for the best organisation of the healthcare systems in our countries.

PART I Political Incentives in Healthcare Systems

I The Political Design of Health Systems

What is the role of the government in healthcare? Can healthcare services be efficiently delivered by markets alone? In a seminal 1963 article, Kenneth Arrow remarked that when economists argue that free markets are able to allocate scarce resources better than any alternative mechanism, they probably do not have healthcare in mind. More precisely, he pointed out that: 'it is clear from everyday observation that the behavior expected of sellers of medical care is different from that of business' (Arrow, 1963, p. 949). He later proceeded by stating: 'it is the general social consensus, clearly, that the laissez-faire solution for medicine is intolerable' (Arrow, 1963, p. 967). Arrow's claims were likely in support of the controversial idea of adopting what would, only two years later, become the first widespread public health insurance scheme in the history of the United States (USA), the joint introduction of Medicare and Medicaid programmes. Arrow's groundbreaking view has had an enduring effect on the health system choices of many different countries around the world.

A simple exercise through which one can appreciate the proliferation of public health insurance schemes (and national health systems) can be conducted by examining cross-country health expenditure trends. Through this exercise, several stylised facts become apparent.

First, as countries become richer, in terms of GDP per capita, total health spending as a share of total GDP increases too (Figure 1.1).[1]

---

[1] This apparent trend has led to debate in the literature over whether healthcare should be considered a normal or luxury good (see Costa-Font et al., 2011a for an empirical account), which has subsequent implications in rationalising a more, or less, ambitious public intervention.

3

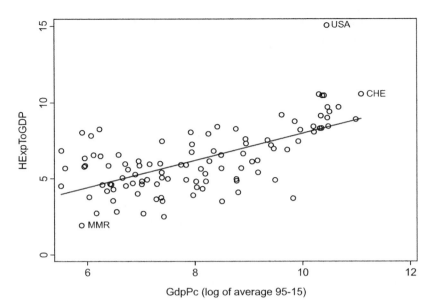

FIGURE 1.1 Health expenditure to GDP (HExpToGDP) correlated with per capita GDP (GdpPc) (average 1995–2015)
Source: Our elaboration from World Health Organization (WHO) data. Sample of countries with more than 4 million population on average for the 1995–2015 period

That is, healthcare is typically a normal good. Both the demand for healthcare and the expectations of better health and quality of care increase with income.

A second, and more salient stylised fact given the focus of this book, is that as countries develop economically, their share of public health spending tends to grow, both in terms of share of total health spending and of total government spending, respectively (Figures 1.2 and 1.3). That is, an expansion of a country's economic development gives rise to an opportunity to widen public interventions in the health sector. We offer a number of explanations which we do elaborate upon throughout this book, among them the expansion of democracy, an instance which comes together with economic development. The central role for the government in healthcare, as we argue below, increasingly situates each individual at the core of the system. Each one of us takes two roles: as a 'patient', interested in obtaining healthcare services of good quality; and as a 'citizen',

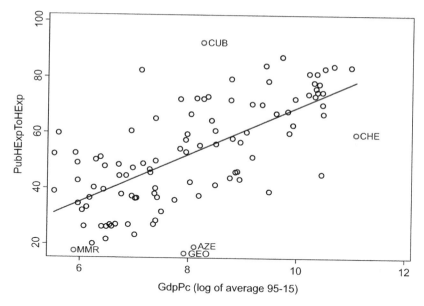

FIGURE I.2 Public health expenditure to total health expenditures (PubHExpToHExp) correlated with per capita GDP (GdpPc) (average 1995–2015)

Source: Our elaboration from WHO data. Sample of countries with more than 4 million population on average for the 1995–2015 period

funding these services and voting for political representatives to legislate on bills shaping health services. These agency relationships between the patient citizen (PC) and the state have progressively become central in the expansion of healthcare activity. Arrow's words have become a self-fulfilling prophecy, as government policy is increasingly at the core of any health system today.

There is a limit to public intervention, as the public financing of the system clearly affects the financial well-being of the PC. That is, insurance premiums, social security contributions or taxes all reduce individuals' income, and hence their consumption of private goods. However, the well-being of the PC increases as the public monies are used to provide quality healthcare services. In our framework, healthcare providers might be a government organisation and/or an independent agent outsourced by the government, as well as market driven private organisations. Some systems are mixed, and allow public and

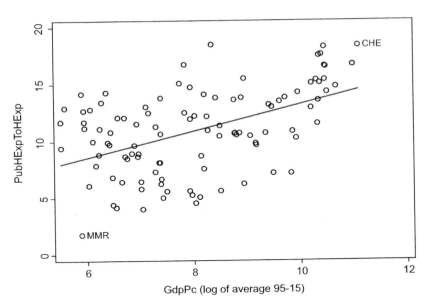

FIGURE 1.3 Public health expenditure (PubHExpToHExp) to total government expenditures correlated with per capita GDP (GdpPc) (average 1995–2015)

Source: Our elaboration from WHO data. Sample of countries with more than 4 million population on average for the 1995–2015 period

private providers to compete, so that market allocations can coexist with equity in the access to healthcare.[2] The implicit assumption here is that the productivity of providers (e.g. such as physicians and hospitals) improves with extrinsic monetary incentives (e.g. a fixed payment per PC treated), but without crowding out other intrinsic motivations, providers naturally have, such as to improve the health and well-being of the PC.[3]

---

[2] In other words, public funding and provision is a way of guaranteeing financial equity, while private provision will stimulates efficiency. This is the idea behind the 'quasi-markets', in which prices are heavily regulated. A variant of these structures when all providers are public is called the 'internal market', as in the UK's reforms in the 1990s.

[3] See, e.g. LeGrand (2002). Whether they work or not as an organisational solution to improve efficiency depends on whether the productivity increase outweighs the transaction costs of operating the market.

Historically, healthcare markets have unfolded in some way or another in almost all countries. They are commonly defined as part of a compact where insurance finances a package of healthcare services. However, when the PC is confronted with the decision about which healthcare providers assure better 'value/quality for money', such judgement is hampered by significant *information imperfections*, as individuals cannot fully judge healthcare quality by themselves. This puts physicians in an advantageous position with respect to the PC (as they can better observe the 'true quality' of care the PC is set to consume). Physicians can either honour their ethical code and become what is labelled as a 'perfect agent' of the PC, or use their informational advantage to pursue alternative courses of action such as induce demand for certain types of healthcare that might, in turn, provide them with additional rents (e.g. Labelle et al., 1994).

A common reaction to the presence of information asymmetries is the *regulation and surveillance of* healthcare, which gives rise to the proliferation of independent agencies that carry out the quality assessment of healthcare services on behalf of the PC. This involves, in many cases, a significant investment in standardising healthcare procedures, for example by developing a taxonomy of treatments that can be classified using Diagnostic Related Groups (DRGs). This allows for instance to adjust the specific case mix of certain providers, and to identify a specific tariff for the public insurer to reimburse each treatment. It also involves developing measures of quality of life such as Quality Adjusted Life Years (QALYs) and other measures of clinical effectiveness, and estimating the value (cost-effectiveness) of different programmes. These designs serve several purposes, including preventing providers from using their private information to maximise the reimbursement they can retain from their medical actions, especially when this might come at the expense of healthcare quality.[4]

Another market imperfection refers to the fact that healthcare contracts are often incomplete, as quality of care and side effects of specific treatment are unobservable to the regulator and the patient,

---

[4] However, their implementation in practice is limited by providers strategic reactions.

and cannot be fully contracted explicitly. As a result, unregulated healthcare markets are not likely to function properly either, which reveals the need for efficient regulation. However, regulation alone might not suffice as special interest groups can develop strategies to lobby regulators and, when opportunities emerge, influence regulation in ways that might not benefit the PC (such as corruption). Hence, monitoring government activity is also necessary to protect the well-being of PCs. Approaches that ignore the latter, and assume that government is perfectly aligned with the interests of the PC, are unrealistic. In real life, health systems, political parties, bureaucrats, lobbies and voters, to mention a few, all play a role in influencing the policy process in the pursuit of specific private goals. Some of those processes might be (and generally are) in conflict with public welfare (Buchanan and Tullock, 1962; Mueller, 1976; Buchanan, 1986).

The pursuit of the private interest in the political arena depends on the design of efficient institutions, or as in North's (1990b) terminology, the rules of the game in a society. Institutions make a significant contribution to constraining the actions of the different stakeholders in the health system. Consider for instance the case of healthcare reforms that require the constitutional approval of two chambers elected under different procedures. This opens up the potential for veto by one of them, which can produce a 'joint decision-making trap': no decision is frequently reached given the significant consensus necessary. However, whether the latter reduces the probability of reform, and guarantees that decisions align with the wider preferences of the constituents, depends on the capacity of agents to reach out to other parties and form cross-party agreements. In advanced democracies, one typically finds processes of logrolling (Stratmann, 2004); that is, transversal exchange of votes between agents that have a veto role, which helps at times to overcome such political impasse. When such exchange is not possible, reforms might not take place or might require amendments. Broader constitutional designs can explain why some health insurance designs are not easily exportable internationally.

Broadly speaking, this book studies the role of institutions and their underpinning political incentives in influencing health and health care. That is, we study of how different institutional designs affect the attainment of socially desirable outcomes such as good health, a more equitable distribution of well-being, an efficient allocation of health resources, and the highest possible quality of care. All these objectives can be obtained (missed) by successfully aligning (or not) political decision-making with the preferences of the PC, the individual at the core of this book. Our definition of 'political economy' is inspired by Buchanan and Tullock (1962). They define 'political economy' as 'the study of the political organization of a society of free men' (p. 3). Although the discipline of political economy is more than two centuries old, it has exhibited significant transformations over time. And as government activity and regulation has made inroads into the health sector, including matters regarding access to healthcare and health finance, the political economy of healthcare has become a central area of study for scholars interested in health policy and practice.

GOVERNMENT INTERVENTION AND THE HEALTH SYSTEM

A healthcare system refers to the organisation of individuals, resources and stakeholders that delivers and finances healthcare needs. It involves interrelationships between payers of healthcare, providers of medical goods, devices and services and, of course, patients and their families as well as the government. This includes the institutional framework in which all implicit and explicit contracts emerging between actors are cast (see Figure 1.4). However, one can contemplate different institutional designs depending on the role of the government and the institutions in place. Even when the government does not directly provide nor fund healthcare, governments play a role in influencing individuals health as they might regulate and tax unhealthy behaviours, or might license new drugs and accredit new hospitals. Such interventions are grounded in authority and compulsion and tend to be motivated by political incentives raising government revenues and exerting authority over industries. More recently, governments design the default options and nudges to attain some of those goals.

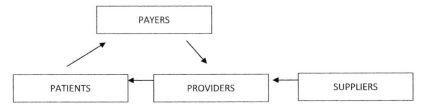

FIGURE I.4 Defining healthcare systems

A Fully Private Market for Services

When insurance markets are not developed, one commonly observes two markets defining the provision of healthcare, namely, one where a private provider delivers healthcare services to patients in need in exchange for a user fee, and a second one where providers (such as hospitals) buy the medical devices and medicines they need to produce such service. This situation is still common nowadays in some sub-Saharan African countries. In these countries most healthcare spending is privately funded and the role of insurance companies is fairly limited.[5] Table 1.1 indicates that in Nigeria private health expenditure accounts for roughly three-quarters of the total, and households are subject to user fees. Out-of-pocket payments by households were as high as 95 per cent of private spending in 2008: back-of-the envelope calculations suggest that 72 out of 100 naira (the local currency) spent in buying healthcare services are paid directly out-of-pocket from households.

Consider now two markets: a market for healthcare services and a parallel market for medical supplies (e.g. drugs, medical devices). If these were two competitive markets (not facing market failures), efficient allocations would arise without a role for the state beyond framing the rules of the game where markets operate. The fundamental

---

[5] Almost all real-world cases are characterised by mixed models, where private funding is used together with public funding to cover healthcare spending. The differences across models are in the relative importance of these two components of funding, as well as in the relative importance of the insurance market in covering healthcare risks with respect to direct out-of-pocket payments.

Table 1.1 *Healthcare financing in some sub-Saharan countries*

Country	Ghana		Kenya		Nigeria		Tanzania		Uganda	
Year	1995	2008	1995	2008	1995	2008	1995	2008	1995	2008
General government health expenditure (GGHE) (% of total)[a]	38.9	49.7	42.7	37.4	21.7	24.7	40.1	65.6	29.4	22.6
Private health expenditure (PvtHE) (% of total)[b]	61.1	50.3	57.3	62.6	78.3	75.3	59.9	34.4	70.6	77.4
GGHE as % of general government expenditure[c]	8.1	7.6	6.3	7.1	7.1	6.5	9.1	16.2	10.1	10.3
Social security funds as % of GGHE[d]	0.0	37.4	11.8	9.1	0.0	0.0	0.0	3.2	0.0	0.0
Private health insurance expenditure as % of PvtHE[e]	6.0	5.9	7.6	8.8	2.4	3.1	4.5	10.4	0.3	0.2
Out-of-pocket health expenditure as % of PvtHE[f]	78.9	79.3	79.3	77.3	95.0	95.8	83.5	75.0	78.9	51.0

[a] The sum of outlays by government entities for health which includes transfer payments to households to offset medical care costs as a percent of total health expenditure in the country.
[b] The sum of outlays by private entities for health as a percent of total health expenditure in the country.
[c] The sum of outlays by government entities for health as a percent of the consolidated outlays of all levels of government.
[d] The sum of outlays on health by government-run social security institutions or national health insurance agencies as a percent of general government health expenditure.
[e] The sum of outlays by private health insurance institutions for a basket of benefits provided to contractually or voluntarily enrolled beneficiaries.
[f] The sum of direct payments by households for health as a percent of private health expenditure.
Source: Carapinha et al. (2011)

contribution by Arrow (1963) was to identify the peculiar characteristics of one of these two markets, the market for medical care services, which operates under significantly different rules than other markets. One can envisage at least five characteristics to consider.

First, individual *demand is often irregular and unpredictable*. The use of healthcare is often driven by healthcare need, rather than preferences. For instance, the use of care after an acute myocardial infarction (AMI), a life-threatening condition, is used by economists as a paradigmatic example of biased patient choice. Patients with a heart attack do not typically demand a specific medical treatment, but rather accept what the doctors in the hospital closest to them choose to supply.

A second characteristic is that the *behaviour of agents* is different from that of other markets for whom self-interest is considered as the norm. Using Arrow's words, the behaviour of a physician is 'supposed to be governed by a concern for the customer's welfare which would not be expected of a salesman' (1963, p. 949). Physicians and nurses are generally seen as people with a vocation for their work, meaning that they are intrinsically motivated and not only interested in material rewards (Barigozzi and Turati, 2012) and the same goes for individuals as organ donors (Costa-Font et al., 2013).

Third, patients generally *do not have first-hand experience* before they utilise healthcare. That is, they cannot ascertain the quality of the service even after utilising it, which makes healthcare a 'credence good' and emphasises the importance of trust in the relationship (e.g. Gottschalk et al., 2018). Economists used to say that healthcare services are characterised by asymmetric information on the quality of services.[6]

Fourth, *supply conditions deviate from those observed in competitive markets*. In competitive markets, supply is driven by the

---

[6] Arrow focused originally more on uncertainty than on quality: he suggested that consumers are uncertain about the consequences of a given treatment they have received, and they also know that doctors possess much more information to predict this uncertainty than they do.

return one can obtain from selling pizzas compared to the return obtainable in selling flight tickets. If return is higher in selling pizzas, then supply increases. In the case of medical care, Arrow observes that suppliers have to be licensed, which restricts supply and increases the costs of production. One can observe that restaurants and airlines are also subject to entry restrictions, but demand for pizzas and tickets do not share the same characteristics as the demand for medical care (e.g. imperfect information). More generally, the limited comparability of health care quality makes healthcare exceptional.

Fifth, the medical profession employs *sector-specific pricing practices*, and carries out extensive price discrimination based on income. The extreme situation includes the delivery free of cost to those patients that are unable to pay by humanitarian organisations such as Médecins Sans Frontières (MSF), which is present in Nigeria in the two poor states of Borno and Yobe. Such unique practices are adopted by charity organisations in many European countries, examples of which are the Bambino Gesù and the Gemelli Foundation in Rome, offering highly complex treatment to poor children from poverty-stricken countries around the world. This is possible because production costs are financed partly by time donations of voluntary physicians and nurses, and money donations by contributors. This is because, generally speaking, people care about the health of others, and individuals are sensitive to inequity and unfairness (Costa-Font and Cowell, 2019).

The above-mentioned features of the healthcare sector exert significant consequences on market outcomes, as already pointed out in Arrow (1963). In the medical care markets, it is possible to identify non-marketable commodities, such as the consumption of certain types of treatments (vaccines) for communicable diseases; inequalities in the access to health facilities for people living areas that are scarcely populated (e.g. Perucca et al., 2019); and then, as already noted, it is common to find restrictions to entry on the supply side.

The inability of market mechanisms to ensure access to healthcare irrespective of an individual's capacity to pay have led to the extension of social insurance systems, which are deemed to offer universal coverage when everyone is covered. Universal coverage is defined by the WHO as the ability to ensure 'that all people have access to needed health services (including prevention, promotion, treatment, rehabilitation and palliation) of sufficient quality to be effective while also ensuring that the use of these services does not expose the user to financial hardship'. However, still today, the goal of attaining universal coverage in healthcare services is far from being reached in many countries. This is clear from Figure 1.5, where Nigeria, alongside most sub-Saharan countries, emerges at the bottom-left part of the distribution of the world countries, with a very low share of public spending over GDP coupled with a coverage index

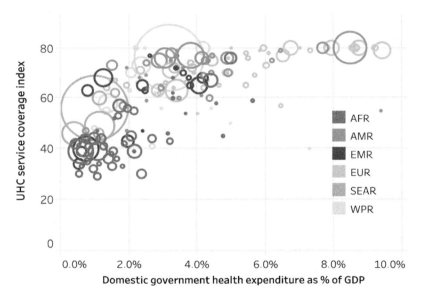

FIGURE 1.5 Public funding and universal health coverage (UHC)
Notes: Data from 2015 or latest available year. Bubble size relative to population. Average coverage of essential services is based on sixteen tracer interventions. Values greater than or equal to 80 are presented as > = 80. AFR = Africa, AMR = America, EMR = Eastern Mediterranean Region, EUR = Europe, SEAR = South-East Asia Region, WPR = Western Pacific Region
Source: WHO (http://apps.who.int/gho/portal/uhc-overview.jsp)

(UCH) below 40 (see Hogan et al., 2018, for all the details related to building the index).

Throughout this book we show that healthcare systems are the outcome of political choices. Such choices are made together with the choice of other institutional designs such as the organisation of multilevel governance and international cooperation; the regulation of the right to healthcare; the expansion of democracy; and the control of corruption and interest groups pursuing goals that do not necessarily align with health improvement and furthering access to healthcare.

As the role of public spending intensifies (and so does the influence of political processes in the allocation of resources devoted to the sector) we observe that the universal health coverage index (see Figure 1.5) first increases and then flattens. The role of political incentives takes centre stage in expanding insurance coverage development, but this is only true until a certain threshold is reached. At some point, spending more public resources does not necessarily imply an improvement in coverage for all, and inequalities remain an open issue. Second, most European countries, alongside the USA and Canada, stand in the flat part of the picture. This evidence already hints that political institutions – like a democratic system of voting – are likely to be important determinants of coverage, not only because public coverage is higher in higher income countries, but also because private markets in these countries are more developed and private insurance markets are better able to hedge health risks. This is clear from Figure 1.6, which maps the relationship between public health expenditure (as a share of GDP) and out-of-pocket spending (as a share of total health spending). The issue of how democracy and its different possible institutions are associated with health and healthcare will be discussed in Part II of the book. As a general observation, it is important to point out that some political institutions help markets flourish; and economic development increases both the public role in the funding of health care (e.g. Greer and Méndez, 2015), and the ability of insurance markets to supply adequate insurance products.

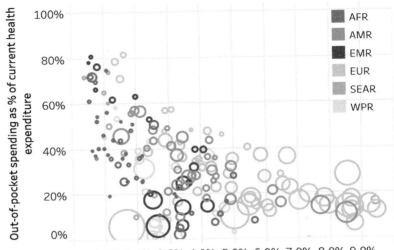

FIGURE 1.6 Public funding and out-of-pocket expenditures
Notes: Data from 2015 or latest available year. Bubble size relative to
GDP per capita. AFR = Africa, AMR = America, EMR = Eastern
Mediterranean Region, EUR = Europe, SEAR = South-East Asia Region,
WPR = Western Pacific Region
Source: WHO (http://apps.who.int/gho/portal/uhc-overview.jsp)

Introducing a Market for Private Insurance

When insurance schemes are introduced, the role of political incentives takes a different course of action. An illustrative example can be identified in the Igunga district, one of the poorest in rural Tanzania, where in 1996 a Community Based Health Insurance (CBHI) scheme was developed. According to Dror et al. (2016), examples of CBHI are 'local mutual aid schemes that put in place arrangements for mobilizing, pooling, allocating and managing or supervising members' resources for healthcare'. Cooperative solutions to cover social risks are the basis of the modern welfare states in Western countries, but are also the antecedents of more developed insurance markets, especially when demand is still limited. However, they can inhibit further government action, and often provide limited coverage.

Historically, economic development has stimulated the development of insurance markets, as well as the expansion of diverse insurance contracts and coverage types. However, as suggested by Arrow (1963), insurance markets are plagued with important market failures as well, and can even encompass some inefficiencies. First, adverse selection arises when only individuals that are more likely to use the health system seek coverage. In this case, unless insurers can differentiate the 'high' from the 'low' risks, insurance will not be viable.[7] As a result, some form of government mandate to have insurance is in place in many Western countries. Second, individuals might change their behaviours regarding the use of healthcare when covered by insurance, and physicians might adopt different clinical practices when they are aware that patients are insured. In these cases, a moral hazard problem could arise, which means that prices and expenditures are likely to be underestimated, and hence insurance contracts will be inefficient. However, so far evidence of demand-side moral hazard is limited as healthcare is more often than not an undesirable consumption unless individuals are in need.[8] In contrast, the literature identifies significant evidence of provider moral hazard. Although moral hazard affects any type of insurance, both public and private, governments limit overconsumption by adding additional rationing mechanisms such as waiting lists and waiting times, which act as an implicit (non-monetary) cost. Avoiding waiting lists and times can give rise to a market for complementary and supplementary insurance, to increase the quality of care on those dimensions in which public systems fall short (Besley et al., 1999).

The USA is one of the outlier countries in that half of the population relies on private insurance, which is mostly employment purchased. The other half is uninsured or covered by some form of

---

[7] Insurers will lose money because insurance premiums typically are set at a level that does not fully reflect the actual characteristics of those who demand insurance.

[8] In addition, part of the increase in consumption after insurance uptake stems from the income effect that results when individuals do not need to pay directly for healthcare (Nyman, 2004).

public insurance either for people over sixty-five (Medicare) or those whose wealth is below a state-specific threshold (Medicaid). However, the existence of public insurance schemes in the USA proves that even mostly private systems require some form of public intervention to address potential market failures, namely the inability to insure those who cannot afford care, and also those that are too old (with a higher probability of falling ill and using medical services that insurers have to then reimburse). However, a significant share of the population still today goes without insurance and healthcare bills are among the main causes of bankruptcy.

The expansion of the population with insurance coverage in the USA has been the result of incremental reforms that have entailed major political manoeuvring to progressively extend insurance coverage. The introduction of Medicaid and Medicare (initially part of the John F. Kennedy and Lyndon Johnson manifestos) were fiercely opposed. Similarly, the most recent insurance expansions, the Afford-able Care Act (ACA), the so-called Obamacare has been at the core of the political debate. The ACA introduced an insurance mandate and a system of individual specific subsidies to make private insurance affordable (insurance exchanges). In addition, it encompassed the design of subsidies to each US state to extend Medicaid entitlement beyond its current threshold. However, such reform has been an object of political opposition by some parties (e.g. constitutional appeals, and repeal proposals by the following administration), as well as by some states (e.g. Texas) given the federal nature of the US health system.[9] Contentious issues were both its cost as well as the compul-sory nature of insurance, which is the standard recipe health econo-mists would have advocated as a way to deal with adverse selection. However, the ACA did pass the two houses, and manage to reduce the share of the uninsured population in the USA. Figure 1.7 shows that the two main periods of reduction of the uninsured population are the

---

[9] Paradoxically, the Republican Party opposing the ACA supported a similar reform that had already been implemented by the Republican Party in Massachusetts.

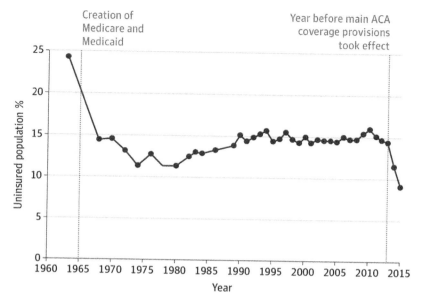

FIGURE 1.7 Percentage of adults without insurance (1960–2015)
Source: Obama (2016)

early 1960s with the introduction of Medicaid and medicare, and the early 2010s with the introdcution of the ACA. The implementation of the ACA has kept the uninsured in the range of 10 per cent. All of these instances point to an important role of the state in the funding of healthcare even when private markets and individual choice play a significant role in resource allocations.

Public Insurance Models

Systems based on insurance choice without a mandate fail to ensure universal access to healthcare, and even when they do, it is common that health systems give rise to what is generally known as a 'two-tier' system with a generous insurance for those who pay privately, and an underfunded insurance scheme for the rest. The latter has led some countries to revert to a fully public model. Publicly funded health systems can be classified as systems where there is a mainstream insurer (a 'single-payer system'), which can be organised either in the form of a National Health Service (NHS) and funded by general taxation (the Beveridgean model), or alternatively be funded by payroll taxes, allocated to a number of independent organisations, so-called sickness funds (the Bismarckian model). In NHS systems, such as in Nordic countries, the United Kingdom (UK), Spain, Italy and Ireland, the government has a large influence in the health system decision-making and the PC has a limited choice of insurance and provider. In contrast, Bismarckian systems generally offer a larger choice of insurance to their beneficiaries, and, as a result, a significant share of healthcare costs is devoted to administrative costs, which means, on average, higher government expenditures in healthcare. However, in such systems, it is common for citizens to exert a political choice in health policy making, especially in federal and decentralised systems, which we discuss in Chapter 2.

Nonetheless, the standard health system classification has become more blurred over time. Whilst Bismarckian systems are mainly funded by social insurance contributions, over time general taxes are increasingly being used to fund healthcare. In contrast, NHS systems traditionally designed to offer uniform care and limited choice, have progressively opened up to devolve responsibilities to subnational tiers of government, and to allow for choice and competition between providers under the assumption that 'money follows the patient'. For instance, hospitals and general practitioner (GP) practices were given budgets to manage (GP fundholding) in the UK under conservative governments, and patients were provided with more choice by the subsequent New Labour government. Originally inspired by the USA, the model was exported to other NHS systems such as Spain and Italy. NHS systems have been, in turn, increasingly decentralised, which provides an additional source of competition (we come back to this point in Chapter 2). Finally, in publicly funded health systems the PC is generally allowed to supplement public healthcare coverage with the purchase of insurance, which mainly lets individuals bypass waiting lists or have access to amenities. Some countries have developed a market for either complementary (such as in France, to cover cost-sharing), supplementary (Spain or Italy) or substitutive private insurance (in Germany, for those above an income threshold), which provides full coverage or direct care for programmes that are not offered in full by the health system, or a more personalised care for services that are offered (Costa-Font and Jofre-Bonet, 2008). Substitutive insurance, unlike the other types of private health insurance, allows for the opting out of the pool of more affluent individuals who tend to be healthier on average (Mossialos and Thomson, 2004).

FROM MARKET FAILURE TO GOVERNMENT FAILURE IN HEALTHCARE

Given the trends outlined in the previous section, an increasing body of research has progressively focused on examining *institutional designs* in the healthcare system organisation, and more specifically understanding when and how government intervention should take place. For instance, some insurance and drug pricing designs are more prone to 'regulatory capture'[10] than others, but not all insurance designs are possible in every country, as ideological and cultural constraints limit the possibility of transferring policies from one country to another.

This book intends to be a starting point for inquiry in a field that, given the importance of healthcare in the public sphere, is still underdeveloped. This is one of the first contributions in this direction. Other partial contributions include Kifmann (2009) and Tuohy and Glied (2013). However, Kifmann (2009) is mainly focused on electoral political and median voter approaches to health, which we cover in Part II of the book. Tuohy and Glied (2013) is a very extensive contribution in coverage but does not include issues around government failures, which are centre stage in this book.

Standard claims about government involvement in healthcare can be grounded on the basis of the more general claims discussed above. Healthcare markets, as other types of markets, are imperfect

---

[10] Regulatory capture occurs when powerful lobbies successfully stir regulations towards their own interests instead of the interests of the public, be it interpreted as consumers, ordinary citizens or voters. We discuss this in detail in Chapter 9.

and hence exhibit market failures. Examples include failures which are often relatively easy to detect as they result from problems of asymmetric information, such as problems of adverse selection, the unravelling of insurance markets, the mistreatment or overtreatment of patients, the presence of public goods (e.g. fluoridation) and externalities (e.g. vaccination). In such a setting, markets tend to fail at allocating resources as they under- or overprovide. One could then claim that government regulation can influence market equilibrium in order to make it closer to what would be expected under no information imperfections.

However, government is generally far from a 'benevolent' and 'omniscient'. Political decision makers can be thought of as rational actors (Buchanan, 1986), who might be well disposed in pursuing the good of the people, but often lack the right political incentives to do so, or the necessary information, or more likely both. In short, self-interested market agents tend not to be very different versions of themselves when involved in making political decisions.[11] Consequently, knowledge and agency problems, often attributed to market failures, are also at the source of what we call government failures.

THE RISE OF THE 'PATIENT CITIZEN'

The progressive development of public intervention in healthcare has given rise to a specific type of parallel agency relationships, the agent of which we refer to in this book as the patient citizen (PC). The PC might need healthcare at some point in the near or distant future and, in addition, is also a citizen of the government that legislates and regulates healthcare services. That is, the PC pays taxes – or a social insurance contribution of some kind – which we refer to as T_i, and expects some given level of quality adjusted care, Q_i, financed with her taxes. Typically, the combination of what patients pay and receive, $W_i = Q_i/T_i$, is what the literature refers to as 'Wicksellian

---

[11] One way to address this problem is that individuals might well adopt different motivations in making decisions depending on their context, and more specifically on 'market' (selfish) or 'government' (altruistic) decision-making frameworks (Margolis, 1984).

connections' (or 'tax-prices').[12] One can monitor the health system design to allow for voice and influence to the PC. Similarly, one can deign health care institutions so that the PC can make more accurate Wicksellian connections.

One way to allow for voice and influence is through political institutions. As discussed in Chapter 4, democracy is understood as a mechanism of preference aggregation where citizens play a central role in making public choices, and typically can take place directly (e.g. direct vote on a proposal via a referendum) as in Switzerland, or, as is common practice in most countries, through mechanisms of representative democracy. When proposals are singled out, one can typically identify the group of voters which tilt the balance in favour (or against) a specific proposal, which are commonly referred to as 'median voter', or as we call them here the median PC.

Representative democracies are typically organised along the lines of political representatives (political parties) people vote for.[13] Political parties compete for voters as companies compete for consumers in many markets. They are typically differentiated by their ideological stances (e.g. liberal, socialist, conservative, green, etc.), and the associated narratives, which are country specific insofar as the inception of democracy has been largely different across countries, and hence the historical antecedents and the media play an important role in people's memories, which in turn affect the narratives in place which gives rise to a 'competition of narratives'. Healthcare plays a central part of such ideological clustering, where different parties hold different conceptions of what an ideal health system should be, such as the nature of the coverage of the system (e.g. migrants, employees, citizens, etc.), the extent of provider and territorial competition, the weight of health inequality reduction as a policy goal, as well as the reduction of access barriers, cost-sharing

---

[12] In honour of the work of the political economist Knut Wicksell (1851–1926), who referred to personalised taxes to finance public goods provision.

[13] The number of political parties depends on the specific electoral system in place (e.g. proportional representation tends to produce more political parties than 'first past the post' or systems based on a majority rule).

and prevention. The PC is at the centre of health system reform, and different parties attempt to represent and gather their support.

The PC is not equally critical in all countries. In some countries, healthcare is more at the centre of the political debate than in others. That is, countries differ on whether healthcare is considered a political, or other, matter. Politics, widely speaking, comes into play in a number of different ways. First, for given political institutions, the PC influences political choices by casting votes to parties which meet their priorities and penalises those that do not, where healthcare is a salient, though not exclusive matter. Elected representatives running the government will then influence healthcare decisions via public regulation, the organisation of the direct public supply of services, and especially the public funding of these services. Political incumbents seeking re-election might also influence the very same political institutions in the long run, by attempting legislative and constitutional changes. In all these cases, markets and individual decisions will then be substituted or might be constrained by collective decisions at different levels. This is the political space that we focus on in this book.

THE MOTIVATION OF POLITICAL DECISIONS

Political decision-making, just like market decision-making, is often motivated by specific rewards and interests of different stakeholders conditioned on a number of restrictions, including ideological, regulatory and financial ones. Ideology might thus explain why some public health insurance reforms are feasible in Europe, but not in the United States.[14] Voters and political decision makers can be seen as self-interested agents who are affected by political marketing campaigns which influence their health care system narratives (Shiller, 2017). However, political incentives are unique in that they influence who

[14] Financial restrictions explain why some middle-income countries can afford certain reforms that reduce health inequality which aren't as feasible in low-income countries (Costa-Font et al., 2018).

exerts power, and take many forms depending on the context (e.g. rents, electoral support and re-election, funding for a campaign or a specific organisation, etc.). The influence of such political incentives is so prevalent in healthcare that it can explain why support for healthcare reforms that reach significant consensus in some countries are a contentious matter in others (e.g. Obamacare in the United States). In day-to-day decision-making, political influence determines who to appoint to become members of the boards of regulatory agencies, deciding the specific morphology of the network of public hospitals and where these hospitals should be located, as well as the funding to be dedicated to them. The problem is that self-interested voters and politicians might not make the decisions that maximise social welfare, but rather their own private benefit. That is, when institutional design does not preclude opportunistic behaviours, public intervention opens up to possibilities of capture and additional layers of agency failures. The latter are likely to result in a misallocation of resources (a 'political failure'). Political incumbents might make a decision on whether to open or close a hospital depending on their electoral rewards (a behaviour defined as 'pork barrel' in the literature), which indicates that political allocation of resources might be inefficient and far from responsive to social needs. These political failures may be just as inefficient as the very allocative inefficiency produced by market allocations in that they are insensitive to social need.

Social insurance is likely to be the most efficient way of funding health and long-term care (Barr, 2001). However, one can easily build a political narrative around the 'primacy of choice' as a halt to social insurance development. Indeed, Cutler and Johnson (2004) explore a number of determinants of social insurance including the strains of capitalism; the need for political legitimacy; the desire to transfer to similar people; increased wealth; and the outcome of Leviathan government. When these types of decisions are generalised, the allocation of healthcare resources is likely to be inefficient. In such a situation, social insurance emerges as a 'second-best' allocation, that is, allocation far from social optimum but that emerge as feasible alternatives, when the optimum is unachievable. But the choice between different second-best allocations in such cases is determined by non-conventional market criteria, and requires the understanding of social, historical, legal and more generally political influence in health decision-making. Addressing the latter is broadly the role of the political economy of health and healthcare.

Finally, we focus on the so-called microeconomic side of political economy (Merlo, 2006) which refers to understanding voters and consumers of healthcare, the policy and political process, but also how the institutions of a country, starting by its constitution, the objectives of its decision makers (most primarily its political elites) and political parties, interest groups and bureaucrats give rise to specific equilibrium outcomes.

THE BOOK'S ROAD MAP

This book is structured in four parts and ten chapters. Rather than embarking into exhaustively reporting a comprehensive survey of all the issues one would expect to find in an 'applied' political economy or public choice textbook, we have addressed in a systematic but non-exhaustive way what we believe are the most important questions on the growing field of the political economy of health and healthcare. Most of these issues are theoretically argued, but more importantly supported by evidence mostly from studies in the area of health economics and health policy. Our intention has been to write a manuscript which is only a first edition, to keep updating to extend in at least two directions. First, to include those questions that could not be covered here, and second, to add evidence and insights that we did not manage to include in this edition.

The current structure of the book is as follows: first we provide an introduction to the key concepts of political economy and why politics comes into play in healthcare. Chapter 1 has defined what we mean by the patient citizen (PC) which is the key agent we focus on, and her preferences. We do not look at the preferences of the PC as an individual, but at her policy preferences in healthcare. Given that voting is at the centre of any democracy, the participation of citizens – who are either current or potential patients – is a fundamental input influencing the political process in democratic health systems. Voters' consent and preferences can be regarded as the 'most fundamental primitive' of political economy models (Downs, 1957a). The second and third parts of the book consider how the PC delegates policymaking to elected representatives at different jurisdictional levels, as well as more generally, how the operation of political competition takes place, and especially, when and how do constitutional prerogatives and ideologies influence the type of decisions that are taken.

More specifically, as we describe in Figure 1.8, the second part of the book (Chapters 2 and 3) focuses on *where (at which level of government such as local, national, international) are decisions made*, or not made (when there are collective action failures). This entails understanding how government adapts its health policies to citizens' heterogeneous needs and preferences at the local level, and when does cooperation for collective action at the global level. A third part

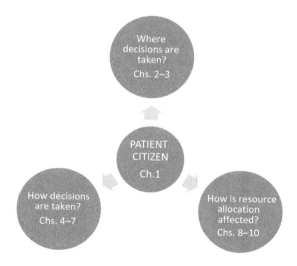

FIGURE 1.8 The questions the book attempts to address

(Chapters 4–7) is devoted to examine *how are healthcare decisions taken* (see Figure 1.8), which means studying how the PC manages to influence health policies and institutions. Finally, the fourth and last section (Chapters 8–10) of the book is devoted to examining questions around 'resource allocation' (how specific forms of political markets influence the allocation of resources), which entails examining waste and corruption, the role of special interests and lobby activities, how voting exchanges take place (logrolling) as the temporal inconsistencies of the political process which influence the weight of healthcare innovation.

Broadly understood, this book conceptualises policy and institutions in the health sector as the result of equilibrium decisions. Such equilibrium comes out of a demand for policies[15] and institutions (so called the 'demand side'), which is revealed by the PCs voting behavior. The PCs preferences are in turn influenced by the media and/or lobbies themselves. For instance, the PC can influence the health system by restricting lobbying, as well as exerting collective action during campaigns and demonstrations. Throughout the book, we will characterise the influence of the PC in different ways, including when it acts as a median or pivotal voter, when the middle-class PC captures the health system, as well as when it forms a coalition of the extremes against the middle class or give in to the demands of lobbysts and rent-seekers. In contrast, the supply side refers to any action that responds to those policy demands, including actors who can legislate on healthcare policies. Finally, the equilibrium defines the policies implemented given the existing constraints which include the electoral rules defining the median voter, or ends-against-the-middle strategies, the constitutions that define the horizontal (executive, legislative and judiciary) and vertical

---

[15] We define the demand side as any actor that demands any new healthcare policies including lobbies, public hospitals. For instance, hospitals, nurses and doctors organise themselves to exert collective action and would be part of the demand side, namely they are interest groups; the same applies to lobbies.

(between jurisdictions including supranational and subnational) power-sharing in a country, the government types (parliamentary or presidential), as well as the dynamics of parties, trade unions and agents influencing the policy process. These should be allocated in the equilibrium as first-order choices that would require a large majorities to change.

Table 1.2 provides a road map that explains the organisation of the different chapters from a supply and demand perspective. Implicit in our argument is that health care institutions result from equilibrium solutions to health policy problems. Such solution are constrained by the way politicians are elected, and policies are selected, the specific role of veto players, the way power-sharing takes place and is implemented and influenced by special interests or bureaucrats. In characterising equilibrium institutions, one can distinguish first-level choices which affect 'basic institutions' such as a country constitution which defines how power is shared, and 'second-level choices' which refer to day-to-day decisions on healthcare reform.

Table 1.2 *The demand and supply of health policies and institutions*

Demand-side factors (election)	Equilibrium	Supply-side factors (selection)
Voters, public opinion and voting	*Constitutional provisions* (first-level choices) such as including federalism model and power division.	Politicians' ideology and partisanship Global collective action
Special interest groups: lobbying and rent-seeking	Policy actions and regulations (second-level choices): including those resulting from logrolling, waste, corruption	Healthcare providers and agencies (administrative rules)
Corporations' regulatory capture		Committees, industrial organisation of Congress

Finally, the prevalent ideology is typically chosen by parties that participate in the supply side of health policies, to distinguish themselves from other competitor parties. In choosing those policies, they limit the political choice set of policy options the PC can choose from.

The first part of the book, this chapter, has defined the key concepts and approaches that define what we refer to as the political economy of health and healthcare. The focus has been on the agency relationships that define the patient citizen. Next, Part II of the book is made up of two chapters examining the jurisdictional level of political decision-making in healthcare, and more specifically the multilevel nature of healthcare decision-making and the collective action challenges of global health *policy*. Chapter 2 examines how decentralisation, and more generally the 'federalisation' of a health system, intersects with healthcare policies in many different countries. Health policies are unlikely to be well managed only at the central level. However, there are clearly some responsibilities more efficiently managed at a higher level of government. The most striking example is public health, which includes confronting the effect of pandemics. This brings us to examine the role of a global governance in healthcare in Chapter 3. This entails not only examining the effect globalisation has on health systems (for example how the expansion of international mobility of patients and providers is reshaping national health systems), but also whether a global governance of healthcare is possible.

Part III of the book discusses in much more detail the mechanisms that explain the rise of the PC. Particularly, Chapter 4 discusses the constitutional design of health systems and the articulation of political power-sharing, and how some constitutional rights (e.g. universal access to healthcare) might be at the expense of other health system goals. Chapter 5 provides an overview of the empirical literature to date on how democracy and democratic transitions influence health. We then discuss what kind of political equilibrium would likely emerge in democratic regimes, including the role of the median voter. Finally, Chapter 7 delves into the role of ideology in shaping both the demand and supply of healthcare policies.

Part IV of the book is devoted to the *analysis of the inefficiencies* in healthcare. In Chapter 8, reviews the sources of waste in healthcare spending and pays special attention to corruption as a source of waste. Next, in Chapter 9, the discussion turns to regulatory capture and rent-seeking activities, as well as lobbying for health policies. Specifically, we discuss the role of special interests in health policymaking and whether competition among such interest groups is ever efficient. Finally, the book ends with Chapter 10, which takes up the issue of innovation in healthcare reform, and how innovation is affected when incentives are distorted by political decisions.

PART II The Political Contexts of Healthcare Policies

2 The Multilevel Nature of Healthcare Governance

THE PURPOSE OF HEALTHCARE GOVERNANCE

Decision-making in healthcare is typically delivered and run by different levels of government. That is, the locus of political decisions tends to be scattered vertically between local, state and supranational powers, in multilevel governance structures. These structures (with a central and subcentral tiers of governments) require a well-informed patient citizen (PC) who is able to judge how well each level of government has managed its responsibilities. As we argue below, if this is the case, the PC will be able to reward successful innovation in health policy by re-electing the incumbent, or by "voting with their feet" to another jurisdiction that exhibits better healthcare performance. We contend that the PC will typically attempt to change the health system on a first instance through the political mechanisms in place, whilst mobility (Tiebout, 1956) is conceived as a last resort option. This chapter describes some of the main issues guiding multilevel health governance, and specifically the difficulty in dealing with the needs of centralising, and decentralising decisions related to global health problems which produce large effects beyond countries' borders (what economists call spillover effects). This includes examining how best to organise a health system between local and central levels within countries. This is the case in legal federations, like the USA or Germany. But it is also the case in regional countries, like Italy or Spain, and also in unitary states, like the Nordic European countries, where municipal governments are the subnational entities. For the purpose of this chapter, we will generalise the observed variety of institutions by using neutral terms like 'central government' and 'subnational governments', and government interactions between them are generally regarded as 'multilevel governance'.

Multilevel governance is important when, as in the case of healthcare, there might be different preferences across jurisdictions on what each government should do (different PC preferences), and on how well it performs on visible dimensions. Take as an example the organisation of primary care or the authorisation of the development of a new paediatric hospital. Both are examples of decisions best made with local knowledge at the local level, whether municipal, provincial or regional, and call for some decentralisation of healthcare policy. The presence of several authorities explains the emergence of multi-level governance, which in different countries adopts the form of 'decentralisation',[1] 'devolution' or 'federalism' (Costa-Font and Greer, 2013; Marchildon and Bossert, 2018).[2]

What is specific to multilevel governments is the existence of intergovernmental interactions between central and other subcentral governments, in turn have overlapping responsibilities.[3] Interactions can take the form of competition or cooperation. As long as each level pursues its goal, interactions have to be understood as strategic moves to obtain the best outcome for each level of government. The available strategies are constrained by the constitutional design of what central and subcentral tiers of government are allowed to do. That is why – as we argue below – the outcomes of decentralisation widely differ across countries.

---

[1] Decentralisation, as defined here, should be considered as a proxy for autonomy of subcentral governments (Oates, 1985), or as a measure of the strength of subnational political power in the form of independent controls on employment, as well as control of regulatory and taxation powers.

[2] Baicker et al. (2012) documents that most of the devolution of public policy responsibilities in the USA takes place in the area of healthcare, which requires complex managerial operations, as well as the design of federal grants to encourage state actions towards efficiency and innovation.

[3] Costa-Font et al. (2014), which provides a metaregression analysis of all the studies documenting intergovernmental interactions, finds that interactions are stronger at local and national level, rather than regions.

When the system of governance is multilevel, it entails a redefinition of the political agency with the PC. In an ideal system, the PC should be able to determine, at each level of government, whether healthcare actions are worth the taxes allocated. As a result, an increase in taxes or expenditures in one state produces spillover effects on neighbouring states at the same level of government (horizontal interactions). A similar effect is produced across different levels of government (vertical interactions).[4]

WHY DO COUNTRIES DECENTRALISE THEIR HEALTH SYSTEM?

Many European countries such as Italy, Spain, and the UK exhibit some level of health care decentralisation. In addition, some health systems are descentralised by design in federal states as in Germany, Switzerland, the US and Belgium. Although health care federalism tends to be more common in high-income countries such as the USA, Switzerland, Germany and Canada, it is possible to list a number of mid-income countries like Mexico, Brazil and South Africa, as well as lower-income countries such as Pakistan, India and Nigeria that have federalised its health system. Hence, it appears that the most pressing question to examine is: what drives countries to decentralise their health system?

Decentralisation is naturally a process aimed at embracing citizens' differences in needs and preferences across the territory without splitting the health system geographically. When heterogeneity is too large a 'one size fits all' health system can become inefficient. Yet, whether decentralisation is desirable or not, boils down to whether the gains from providing heterogeneous policies across local constituencies overcomes the higher costs from a decentralised provision of healthcare services (resulting from not taking advantage of the lower

---

[4] This is typically the case, whether the state is formally federal or not (Breton and Fraschini, 2003; Costa-Font and Rico, 2006a).

economies of scale, and higher transactions costs compared to a centralised health system) both PC's (Oates, 1972).

In a descentralised health system, if preferences and willingness to pay for different health programmes differ across jurisdictions, then individuals can 'vote with their feet' à la Tiebout, 'exiting' their jurisdiction, and either choosing healthcare out of their constituency or deciding to reside in an area where their preferences for healthcare match the existing supply. When mobility is too costly, citizens can exercise their 'voice' by electing the opposition government provided they are supplying policies closer to their preferences. These two mechanisms, 'exit' and 'voice', help explain the presence of internal patient mobility based on observable quality differences across providers, both between regions and within each region (see, for the case of Italy, Levaggi and Zanola, 2007; Fabbri and Robone, 2010; Perucca et al., 2019).

There are significant limitations for the average PC, even if well advised, in identifying a place where the quality of care is higher, and exert made use of the exit option. Sharing information on hospital quality among friends and colleagues who have experienced care, might mislead patients (e.g. Moscone et al., 2012). Also, the costs of mobility within a given territory might be too high to compensate for the potential benefits regarding many procedures, unless perhaps very specialised services.

By increasing the centres of political decision-making, decentralisation is also likely to give rise to a number of veto players which can also slow down central-level legislation, and coordinated action when most needed. However, decentralisation can allow regions or states to legislate at their jurisdictional level without waiting for central level consensus. Veto players tend to preserve the status quo, as the consensus required for change to take place makes it much harder to happen. More importantly, decentralisation can give rise to competition between central and subcentral authorities. Piperno (2000) and Montolio and Turati (2017) report that in Italy and in Spain (two countries where regions concur with the central government to legislate on healthcare matters), conflicts between the central and the regional governments are quite common. For instance, the national parliament still rules on decentralised responsibilities and the regional government is frequently opposed to change. Similarly, the central government frequently vetoes regional laws which lead to 'constitutional conflicts of competence' that tend to be ruled in favour of central governments, as the members of the Constitutional Court are directly or indirectly appointed by national parliaments.[5]

Probably one of the most advocated arguments in favour of decentralisation refers to its role in incentivising experimentation and new policies, which takes place without waiting for a country-wide majority support. An example can be found in the introduction and prioritisation of mental health policy in a handful of Spanish regions (Costa-Font et al., 2011b). On the other hand, one of the most cited potential costs of a decentralised health system lies in the allocation of its fiscal responsibility. The higher the share of subnational spending is financed with transfers from the centre, the more subnational governments' budget constraints become 'soft', the higher the spending and deficits at the subnational level (Bordignon and Turati, 2009; Crivelli et al., 2010). Below we will elaborate on some of this points by distinguishing political and fiscal spaces.

THE FISCAL AND POLITICAL SPACE

Decision Space

A recurrent finding is that most federations are characterised by 'centralising tendencies', mostly through direct intervention by the central government framework legislation (e.g. 'basic health laws') that limits the responsibility of subnational authorities and increases the space of the central government. For instance, in Mexico, restrictions exist on the funding allocation to human resources, medicines,

---

[5] This feature is what we refer to as vertical competition below, which, as we argue, when well designed can lead to an expansion of the efficiency of the health system.

public health and infrastructures; in contrast, in Brazil, the similar laws allow the invasion of subnational government responsibilities (Marchildon and Bossert, 2018). Even in industrialised countries, such as Germany, the growing role of federal taxes in funding social health insurance increases the decision space of the federal government. Hence, one cannot truly judge the decision space that a federation provides for health policymaking just by looking at legislation. The financing mechanism is a key mechanism to restrict the decision space of subnational jurisdictions. Indeed, the use of conditional block grants is employed in almost every country to limit subnational governments' capacity. This is even the case in rural countries such as Nigeria, where the case for a central-level control seems rather weak. Similarly, subnational governments have considerably more decision space on specific policy areas such as hospital care, and less in other areas that exhibit considerable externalities such as pharmaceutical policy.

The decision space refers both to the ability to tax citizens with locally managed taxes, which is defined as the *fiscal space*, as well as the capacity to set out legislation and veto the legislation proposals of other levels of government, namely the *political space*.

The Fiscal Space

The capacity of each level of government to raise existing taxes and define new ones is generally not an evident feature capable of being identified by the PC.[6] At the core of 'fiscal' federalism (meaning the multilevel division of the power to tax citizens) lies the idea of solving the so-called Samaritan's Dilemma at the territorial level (Buchanan, 1975a). That is, fiscal responsibilities should be allocated to each level of government in order to make sure that budget constraints at the

---

[6] The administrative division of responsibilities among levels of government is an imperfect measure of decentralisation. There have been a variety of indices of decentralisation which we do not review here but that include proxy variables for autonomy, allocation of responsibilities and political accountability. We will come back to this in the next section.

local level are hard rather than soft, so that fiscal resources act as a constraint to healthcare spending and subnational budgets are balanced. However, it is commonly observed that lower levels of government react by running deficits that call for a central level bailout in the short run (the so-called soft budget constraint problem) and might further expand future spending. A system in which each subnational government finances its own healthcare system entirely is not a viable solution, since inequalities in the tax bases will inevitably result in inequalities in the services provided to citizens. To solve this problem, decentralised systems everywhere are equipped with equalisation grants and centrally defined standards of care. Both grants and standards of care are designed to avoid fiscal autonomy being at odds with redistribution of resources, since most federal designs explicitly or implicitly take equity and solidarity as an important goal of the system (Oates, 1999).

The Political Space

A more recent view of how economists see decentralisation is as a way of tightening the political agency between constituents and incumbents to enhance the mechanisms of the so-called political agency (Besley, 2006). It is different from formal (or legal) federalism, in that the former is a constitutional decision whilst the latter is the result of the political bargaining that takes place both before and after the constitution of a country is determined. But it produces comparable effects insofar as it gives rise to inter-jurisdictional interactions, however, only in federal states do states own powers which operate in a similar fashion as property rights in a market, and hence central governments cannot legally take over decentralised responsibilities. As we will discuss later in the text, in unitary and regional states, the central state commonly exerts an active role in invading overlapping responsibilities of regions and states, and in issuing framework laws that can act as an indirect means for limiting subcentral healthcare autonomy.

Most health system designs are the result of negotiations between key stakeholders, and healthcare governance is mostly the reflection of such exchange mechanisms. Multilevel governance divides the political cycle across the territory, and opens the door to competition, both among subcentral health systems to attract constituents, and with central governments for the transfer of further responsibilities and economic resources.[7] In a multilevel polity, the PC can compare some salient dimensions of their regional health service with that of other regions, like for instance the length of waiting lists and waiting times, the size and internal organisation of the bureaucracy and more generally process-related outcomes that might not be related to the adequacy of treatment and other quality of care dimensions. When decentralisation is not available, the failure of the public insurance to satisfy the heterogeneous demands of all social groups can lead to the emergence of a private market for health insurance, and more generally the 'opting out' to the private sector. Conversely, decentralisation by catering to regionally heterogeneous groups in a health system can, satisfy the specific needs of individuals that otherwise would opt out to the private sector (Costa-Font and Ferrer-i Carbonell, 2019).

INSTITUTIONAL IMBALANCES

Vertical Imbalances

There is consensus among scholars that the key to the success of decentralised health systems boils down to its institutional design. If one plots the degree of expenditure decentralisation and the per-capita health spending, the relationship that emerges is far from clear (see

---

[7] See, for instance, the current discussion in Italy on the request by three of the most important and rich regions for additional space of autonomy to the central government, or the tensions originated from similar requests of the Catalan government to the central government in Madrid over the last few years around a fixed co-payment per prescription drugs and, the extension of health care coverage to migrants.

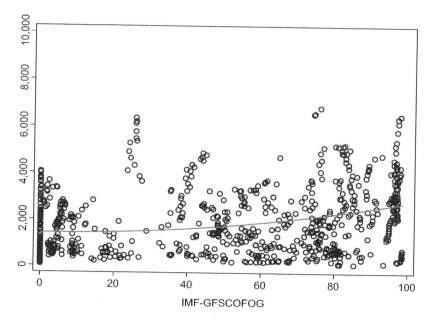

FIGURE 2.1 Decentralisation and total health spending per capita
Notes: Sample of world countries 1995–2015. Y-axis: public health
expenditure per capita, PPP (constant 2011 international $). Source is
World Bank-WDI. X-axis: health decentralisation indices obtained as
(1 - CENTREHEALTHSPEND/TOTHEALTHSPEND) * 100.
Source: IMF Government Finance Statistics, COFOG details (IMF-GSF-COFOG)

Figure 2.1). That is, rather than decentralisation alone, healthcare
spending is influenced by specific multilevel designs.

The extent to which decentralisation manages to align the
political credit for the provision of health care quality, and the
'blame' for any addition tax to be faced by the PC to finance these
services is complex. If the central government fails to shift the
'blame' (due to taxation) to subnational governments and only
decentralises mechanisms of credit-claiming (tax revenues already
collected to spend on health care). It is not surprising that decentralisation naturally results in regional incumbents expanding
healthcare activity (and spending) as they don't bear its political
costs (Costa-Font, 2010b). Similarly, if subnational health

authorities are left with insufficient own resources, this might inhibit innovation and competition, and as a result, the degree of diversification and experimentation in the system. In such cases, one might not observe a generalised efficiency outcome from government decentralisation. One of the most striking problems of decentralised governments lies in the design of incentives for diversity and competition. In doing so there are a set of features that should be taken into account, including the following:

First, budget constraints should not be perceived as being soft, as is the case in some European health systems. An example of social insurance systems reveals that subcentral governments can veto tax increases, but cannot veto social security expansions, which might actually lead to overspending under federalism, as in the case of Germany.

Second, subnational governments must have adequate resources to pursue their activities. If revenues of subcentral governments do not equal or exceed their expenditures, then vertical fiscal imbalances arise. Fiscal imbalances between central and subcentral governments are common both in unitary states and in federations. These imbalances are corrected through the use of transfers, which can be discretionary – and hence politically manipulated – or based on an allocation formula to adjust for differences in needs and risk across subnational governments. However, countries differ as to whether healthcare receives funds according to a specific allocation formula (e.g. adjusted or unadjusted per capita rules), or instead are part of the general funds (including other forms of social spending) that are allocated to subcentral governments. Overall, the more transparent and general the financing of subnational governments, the more it encourages financial planning and efficiency. For instance, the Bartlett formula used in the UK is based on the principle that any increase or reduction in expenditure in England will automatically lead to a proportionate increase or reduction in resources for the devolved governments in the other countries of the UK.

Third, together with vertical imbalances, the effects of governments' actions should not exceed their jurisdictional domain. Another parallel effect is that of the existence of significant disparities in the size and capacity of regional governments, the latter requiring either adjustments for population or risk in the allocation.

Empirical evidence suggests all countries that have decentralised their health system, transfers represent a large proportion of subnational governments' revenues (OECD, 2016). Intergovernmental transfers are viewed as a supplementary means of finance to tackle the existence of negative externalities of some subcentral governments over others (e.g. touristic areas tend to exhibit higher healthcare demand over the summer than neighbouring areas). Transfers act as a source of insurance against region-specific shocks (e.g. epidemics). They are more generally employed to take advantage of the central government economies of scale in tax collection. The obvious downside, which we referred to earlier, is that unless transfers contain fiscal effort corrections, they can lead to soft budget constraints. Indeed, one of the most documented empirical regularities in the fiscal federalism literature is the so-called flypaper effect (Hines and Thaler, 1995; Gamkhar and Shah, 2007). This effect refers to the observed stimulus of unconditional grants on local government spending, which gives rise to an increase in community disposable income.

Horizontal Imbalances

Together with vertical imbalances, the design of federal health systems considers the emergence of horizontal imbalances, such as differences in health outputs between jurisdictions at the same level of government. Such imbalances can emerge primarily as a result of differences in a certain jurisdiction's capacity to provide public services, differences in needs, as well other reasons, like choices and preferences at the local level. Generally, to deal with differences in needs, most federal systems take into account some risk-adjustment criteria in designing equalisation grants thought to compensate for pre-existing differences.

Several studies suggest that regional inequalities in health care activity appears to decline (or not to increase) with decentralisation, though effects on outcomes are rarely identified. Baicker et al. (2012), in their examination of fiscal federalism in the USA, compute the coefficient of variation of several programmes and consistently found that the main programmes that have been devolved to the states exhibit lower regional inequalities. Similarly, in Spain it has been demonstrated that regional inequality in health care activity declined with decentralisation.[8] Importantly, regional inequalities in Spain, where devolution is managed regionally, have decreased by 50 per cent, whilst in the centralised English NHS we see a very modest decline. In contrast, in England, a highly centralised national health system, regional inequalities are more than double those of Spain and have remained stable over time.

How can we explain such a phenomenon? One explanation lies in the effects of equalisation mechanisms and a certain failure in England to deal with region-specific needs and preferences. Whilst this might be true, it does not fully explain why we do not observe the same downward trend in other countries. A second explanation links the influence of policy diffusion as a mechanism to externalise the innovations, whereby traditionally lagging regions import the innovations of front-runner regions, which has been documented in Spain (Costa-Font and Rico, 2006a). These mechanisms would not exist in centralised health systems. Hence, it appears that although decentralisation does indeed allow for diversity in health policies, in the longer run such diversity might well decline in the presence of policy diffusion, and more generally when the mechansims of credit-claiming by innovative governments, become fully operative (Costa-Font and Turati, 2018).

---

[8] See Costa-Font and Rico (2006b) and Costa-Font (2010b).

CHALLENGES

A Race to the Bottom?

Decentralisation can be seen as a means to increase government competition in taxes (and not just in quality) to reduce the size of the state in health care. That is, in a scenario where governments have to run balanced budgets (hence no deficits are allowed in the long term), one would expect a waning of unnecessary expenditures and red tape after government competition. This hypothesis was put forward by Brennan and Buchanan (1980)[9] who predicted that descentralisation would lead to individuals sorting into states based on their policy preferences. This would, in turn, discipline the spending activity of regional incumbents. Alternatively, when one allows preferences to be heterogeneous across jurisdictions, then decentralisation becomes a way to select preferences and policies, rather that to reduce health care investment altogether. Oates (1972) was the pioneer of this counterbalancing argument. In the case of healthcare, empirical evidence is consistent of the second effect, and suggests evidence of a 'race to the top'. Different explanations have been put forward to explain why public expenditure increases after decentralisation:

(i) *Short-term scale economies loss versus long-term efficiency gains.* Health expenditure might increase in the short run but not in the long run as efficiency gains from better sorting of preferences and policies would entail savings for the health system. Consistently with this argument, Costa-Font and Moscone (2008) find evidence that experience in managing healthcare responsibilities gives rise to a reduction in expenditure per capita.

(ii) *Collusion* (Brennan and Buchanan, 1980). Given that regional health systems might be aware of the costs of competition, they might find some explicit or tacit cooperation mechanisms. In addition, many decentralised

---

[9] According to this hypothesis, decentralisation stands out as a pro-competitive mechanism to tame down the Leviathan as follows: 'total government intrusion into the economy should be smaller, ceteris paribus the greater the extent to which taxes and expenditure are decentralised' (p. 15).

health systems are subject to intensive coordination. Finally, the constitutional role of framework laws in Germany, Italy and Spain place a limit on the extent of healthcare experimentation.

(iii) *Vertical competition and policy innovation* can explain, to a certain extent, why a standard race to the bottom does not take place. Competition between central and regional authorities to expand their responsibilities might reduce the incentives to cut down public spending. Costa-Font and Rico (2006a) provide evidence that vertical competition in healthcare has led to a logic of healthcare expenditure expansion. Part of such an effect lies in the fact that vertical competition stimulates policy innovation, as one way to keep responsibilities that can be allocated to several jursidictions has lead to the introduction of new programmes which are supported by the PC. Wallis and Oates (1988) use an alternative explanation for expenditure rise based on the existence of government differentiation which is consistent with findings suggesting policy innovation is boosted to keep the cannibalisation effects of competition under control.

(iv) *Political markets.* Decentralisation brings power closer to the citizenry, and hence enhances political incentives for incumbents to influence policy action in order to guarantee re-election. If the incentives of regional incumbents are not driven by mobility but exclusively through the political agency, then governments will attempt to accommodate the preferences of the median voter to seek re-election. If the median voter tends to support the widening of healthcare coverage, as is the case in many European countries, one would expect that inter-jurisdictional competition would lead to an expansion of the size of the health system.

(v) *Fiscal design.* Finally, an alternative explanation for the absence of a race to the bottom in healthcare lies in the fact that the fiscal design of decentralised health systems relies too heavily on central-level funding, such as block transfers and, in turn, gives rise to a high degree of borrowing autonomy which engenders fiscal deficits (Crivelli et al., 2010), and limit competition. This is the case in the UK with the Bartlett formula.

Voting with One's Feet

A potential source of government competition can take place through patient mobility (Tiebout, 1956). In the United States, 2.5 per cent of residents change state every year. In contrast, mobility is far more limited in Europe for a variety of reasons, including that individuals build significant attachments and networks at the local level, as well as other social barriers, such as linguistic differences, that even take place within countries such as Switzerland and Spain where differences in language can stand as limits to mobility. A similar situation can be found at a European level. Since the 1990s the European Court of Justice has responded with a row of cases granting foreign workers the right to access the guest state's healthcare system, and the patient mobility directive (2011/24/EU) regulates the right to receive non-hospital care in another member state, and ensures patients' free movement in the European Union without pre-authorisation. Reimbursement is based on the fees applicable in the home state of a patient. However, the potential for mobility does not necessarily entail competition, in part because patients are reluctant to travel, and reimbursement regimes might not encourage hospitals to attract non-resident patients. Mobility is common in certain conditions such as cancer care where only certain areas have access to specific health technologies or, when certain technologies are not available, patients are asked to pay privately.

Accountability

One of the main mechanism that explains how decentralisation improves outcomes is the strengthening the political agency of the PC with their own health system decision makers. This is the case when decision makers are responsive to the demands of the PC. The most obvious way to enhance political accountability is through electoral processes at all levels of government so that officials align with the interests of the PC. Elections should be based on subnational government-specific affairs and not intertwined with other country-wide matters, as for instance is the case in many Spanish regions (Costa-Font, 2009). The mechanisms of the political agency imply that individuals as citizens are active agents that learn and make comparisons using evidence from other similar governments to evaluate whether they are getting 'value for money'. That said, as we discuss later in the book, the supply of health policies depends on the role of special interests and lobbyists that influence the political process, alongside pockets of corrupted officials, which often emerge at all levels of government.

Experimentation

Decentralisation is deemed to foster bottom-up experimentation and evolutionary selection of best practices. Indeed, the link between decentralisation and experimentation has been an old argument that dates back to the Hayek (1948) view that decentralisation, by increasing experimentation, produces more information on how to run a government. Healthcare is one of the clearest-cut examples of a laboratory of public policies. The example of the USA shows how the latest federal healthcare reform shares significant knowledge from healthcare reform in Massachusetts. Evidence from different countries reveals that experimentation does take place after devolution for varying reasons. First, junior governments tend to legitimise themselves by introducing and experimenting with new policies (e.g. free long-term care and no prescription charges in Scotland and Wales, respectively). Second, decentralisation can help to nurture some degree of vertical competition with the central government that can provide additional political incentives for innovation (Costa-Font and Rico, 2006a). Finally, if soft budget constraints are corrected, experimentation can provide fiscal incentives for costs savings.

Political Competition

The fiscal federalism literature contends that governments' competition can be welfare-improving (Breton, 1996). The most obvious form of competition comes out of tournaments theory, whereby the PC in one jurisdiction evaluates the performance of their own constituency relative to other jurisdictions (Salmon, 1987). The main downside of such a mechanism is that performances are not easily observable, especially quality dimensions that motivate citizens to either move or use political agency to punish or reward the incumbent party ruling the health system. Finally, a final important question that can be inferred from the litertaure is that of the welfare effects of healthcare decentralisation; they depend quite critically on the success of political competition in incentivising innovation. Consistently, Salmon (2019) argues that devolution does not automatically benefit large and heterogeneous communities. If diversity does not give rise to different policies, decentralisation might just give rise to 'more of the same'.

Local and Country-Level Capture

One of the common concerns on the decentralisation of health policy is that of 'local capture', leading to government failure[10] as discussed in Chapter 9. The argument here is that decentralisation brings local providers and regulators closer, so that if mechanisms of public sector purchasing are not transparent enough, they might lead to the risk of local capture (Laffont, 2000). An important dimension to be considered is whether local lobbies have conflicting interest or not. In the former case, lobbying is less damaging for social welfare under centralisation than under decentralisation. In the latter case, lobbying is less damaging under decentralisation, provided that spillover effects are weak (Bordignon et al., 2008).

SUMMARY

This chapter has provided an overview on a broad set of questions that the decentralisation of health systems brings to the fore. We have examined important design features including how best to address fiscal imbalances, regional inequalities, policy innovation and making sure that the mechanisms of the political agency align individuals' preferences and needs with that of their incumbent's priorities. We have specifically discussed several limits to the success of

---

[10] See Costa-Font and Puig-Junoy (2007) for an example in the Spanish setting.

decentralised health systems, including the alignment of fiscal and political accountability, the design of resource allocation mechanisms that bypass soft budget constraints and more generally the development of incentives to policy diffusion that, if successful, can reduce long-term inequalities.

3 'Collective Action' and Global Healthcare

The effects of health services and interventions increasingly transcend the borders of nations, and our most ambitious challenges today are driven by the pursuit of global health goals. Global healthcare policy includes the supply of health programmes, goods and services that by exceeding the boundaries of nations produce significant externalities (effects to other health systems). Examples include the control and eradication of epidemics, the access to essential medicines of the entire world population and the need to standardise the practices of health professionals to match the 'best practices', when known and available. Hence, it involves decisions around international mobility of healthcare inputs like health technologies, medicines, vaccines and health professionals and their role in promoting global health.

The main political challenge that global healthcare poses is that of solving the problem of collective action. That is, although poverty rates and health indicators in poor countries have undergone tremendous improvements in the last twenty years (Deaton, 2004, 2014), healthcare decision makers are generally reluctant to undertake actions that have a global impact. That is, the pursuit of global health goals is challenged by collective action problems (Olson, 1965; Sandler, 2004). Countries pursuing public health goals that improve the health and welfare of the entire world are subject to strong incentives to free-ride on the endeavours of others. In such cases, global healthcare actions are underprovided unless those countries contributing the most to the supply of the collective good find a way to enjoy specific and selective incentives in doing so. These cases are labelled

Table 3.1 *Categorisation of incentive structures depending on the types of healthcare and disease*

		Healthcare/medicine	
		Curative	Preventive
Disease	Communicable	C. Unclear	A. HGCA: Successful
	Non-communicable	B. HGCA: Problematic	C. Unclear outcome

Note: HGCA = Health Global Collective Actions.

by Olson (1965) as 'privileged' public goods, since at least one of the countries involved in the provision of these global goods enjoys extra private benefits which are higher than the costs of supplying the good alone. Consequently, the reasons for the failures or successes of global collective action in health have to be found by analysing the underlying selective incentives to free ride. The nature and distribution of such incentives are related to the type of healthcare provided – whether curative or preventive – and to the disease at hand – whether communicable or not. This is illustrated in Table 3.1, which categorises the incentive structures depending on the types of disease and care.

More specifically, A in Table 3.1 refers to preventive care, such as a low-cost vaccine that prevents a communicable disease. In this case, the costs of global provision are low and the benefits are high, hence there are enough incentives to carry out global actions given that in such a scenario there are likely potential spillovers to other countries. This explains why the global community has managed to eradicate some health conditions such as smallpox, but no other types of disease (Sandler, 2004). In contrast, B illustrates the case of a high-cost curative treatment tackling a non-communicable disease. Here, the selective incentives are weak, and it is likely that health global collective action will fail. Intuitively, curing a communicable disease is usually cheaper, for example antiretroviral medicine for HIV, and benefits to individual countries are potentially large. In contrast, the cures for a non-communicable disease such as chemotherapy are way more expensive than antiretrovirals or vaccines and do not produce relevant effects on other countries. Finally, there are 'grey zones', as represented by C and D, that have to be evaluated on a case-by-case basis.

This chapter discusses the difficulties in engaging in global health collective action, which is why global health might suffer from potentially severe underprovision. To date, there is no supra-national government authority with full responsibilities for global health. The World Health Organization (WHO) is the United Nations agency specialised in health-related matters, but can only promote coordination among nations. Instead, healthcare decision-making – even when it impacts on global health – is highly decen-tralised and multilateral, depending in some cases on the initiative of single countries. When it takes place, cooperation requires the adherence from several national governments who can opt out of international agreements, or even veto collective action initiatives. Global collective action failures give rise to what is called a global governance 'deficit', or what some call 'global gridlock' (Hale et al., 2013). The multiplicity and fragmentation of stakeholders with dif-ferent interests, the presence of country- and area-specific problems (such as the epidemics specific to poor sub-Saharan African coun-tries, like Ebola) and a potential for institutional inertia (to arrange solutions that entail costs in the short run for some countries) are issues to be considered if one wants to attain a global welfare improvement.

In addition to the limits posed to collective action, global health stakeholders face a potential thread of *regulatory capture*. For example, budgets of big-pharma multinational corporations are now potentially larger than some small countries' GDPs, let lone their health system budgets. Indeed, the 2016 annual report for the top ten pharmaceutical companies suggests that their R&D budgets added up to $70.5 billion[1] whilst in the same year Malta's GDP was $12 billion, Slovenia's was $45 billion and Croatia's was $51 billion. The emergence of corporate power, in turn, partly explains the increasing processes of integration in some parts of the Western world to expand the scale of governments. These large supranational governments are able to more fiercely oppose the power of such international corporations, especially their attempts to lobby governments for favourable healthcare policies and, at times, capture healthcare regulators.

Although global health interventions can be argued to predate the globalisation era (e.g. the rapid spread of worldwide interaction observed after the collapse of the Soviet Union), the growing globalisation of a number of health inputs (e.g. medicines, vaccines, etc.) calls for some form of collective action at that level too. Increasing interdependence reduces the barriers to access healthcare services and information, mobility of patients and providers (given declining transportation costs). This goes along with the development of international institutions that promote free trade, such as the World Trade Organization (WTO). Parallel to this, the development of information and communication technologies has contributed to the spread of health information and knowledge across the world, which has promoted the diffusion of high-cost health technologies as well as best practices in health management procedures globally. These changes have improved access to treatments that were not available before and provided the incentives to reducing local specific bottlenecks in health services. However, global interdependence brings important vulnerabilities and risks to security too, including an increasing exposure to health shocks affecting other countries, as well as limiting the national pricing of new technologies.

---

[1] Fierce Biotech (2017). www.fiercebiotech.com/special-report/top-10-pharma-r-d-budgets-2016.

The remainder of the chapter delineates some of the desirable effects of competition or coordination in global health policy. Whilst cooperation emerges as more efficient in the management of goods characterised by large externalities, international competition would be expected to deliver more efficient allocation of health resources with limited externalities. Examples include differences in prices due to varying supply conditions across countries (for instance, the provision of dental health care in middle- and lower-income countries cost much less, and become more homogeneous with mobility). Similarly, the attraction of healthcare professionals from lower-income countries is typically, at the expense of the needs of such countries. Another example is that of health technologies which are globally launched by multinationals, whilst their regulation and pricing is largely domestic. Hence, healthcare governance operates in a rather different way under economic interdependence (Blouin et al., 2009).

GLOBALISATION AS A NEW CHALLENGE

Global Collective Action for Health

The global interdependence of behaviours, information sources, healthcare inputs, cultures and technologies shapes how health systems are organised. Such a phenomenon is typically referred to as 'globalisation'. In this chapter, we discuss how such interdependence creates a vacuum in global health governance. Most health systems have been organised within the contours of the nation state, and problems that exceed such scale tend to be unaddressed. This is what we referred to earlier as a 'collective action' problem.

The problems of collective action in promoting public health have worsened with the expansion of economic and social interdependence. In the first half of the twentieth century, countries adopted different preventive interventions and best practices in sanitation systems, vaccinations and household behaviour, and were able to manage and control the spread of communicable diseases more effectively. This led to a reduction of mortality rates, especially those of infants and young people, key indicators in measuring human development.[2]

The global collective action problem has been solved for some health interventions, but there are still challenges to overcome. Consistently with Table 3.1, the success in global health policy has mostly occurred in *preventive care*, targeting the containment or eradication of communicable diseases, which has had significant, if not enormous, positive externality effects. It can be argued that part of this was motivated by the self-interest of high income countries to avoid the spread of communicable disease as a sort of self-protection (such as the recent experience with coronavirus in China). Population mobility and, therefore, disease mobility, has increased tremendously with globalisation. This has been a critical *selective incentive* to solve the free-riding problems that limit global collective action. However, disease mobility is accompanied by some critical challenges.

A significant challenge refers to determining how to incentivise the spread of *curative medicine*, which benefits mainly treated individuals and their countries (and are not global public goods). Overcoming this challenge will require increased effort in the diffusion of specific infrastructures (hospitals), managerial skills and high-level know-how on the part of providers, as well as the diffusion of complex practices and technologies. This is particularly important, as the incidence of non-communicable diseases (cancer, cardiovascular diseases, etc.) is also increasing in developing countries.[3]

---

[2] This does not mean that differences across nations have disappeared. The downward trends observed everywhere still leave poor countries largely behind most developed nations. For instance, the World Bank suggests that the under-five mortality rate in Sierra Leone and Mali today is at the same level of Portugal back in 1960. India and Botswana lag behind by about forty years. See *World Development Report 2017* at www.worldbank.org/en/publication/wdr2017.

[3] See here for some data: www.who.int/news-room/fact-sheets/detail/noncommunicable-diseases.

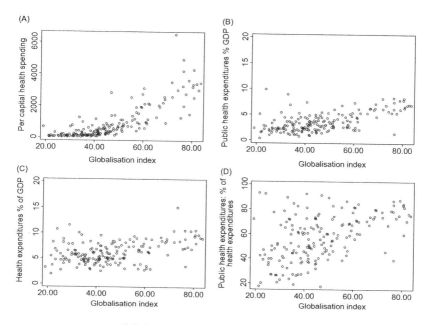

FIGURE 3.1 Globalisation index and health expenditures: (A) per capita health spending, (B) public health expenditures as % of GDP, (C) health expenditures as % of GDP and (D) public health expenditures as % of health expenditures

Regardless of collective action failures, it is possible to find a positive association between measures of healthy life expectancy and globalisation (measuring using the KOF globalisation index). A similar association can be found with other measures of health, like infant mortality which is in part expressing an increasing demand for health, which translates into an induced demand for healthcare. Consistently, Figure 3.1 reveals an association between globalisation and per capita health expenditure measures. More specifically, we document an association between globalisation and the share of expenditure on GDP, as well as the share of public expenditure and total health expenditures. However, such an association is confounded by a number of other effects, including the effect globalisation has on income and poverty and the transmission of health-related knowledge (Deaton, 2004). Similarity, globalisation does encompass speedier circulation of risky health behaviours and connected diseases, such as obesity, that result from the adoption of a Western lifestyle (Costa-Font and Mas, 2016). It can also be a source of new potential vulnerabilities (Amrith, 2001). The adoption of new lifestyles encompasses higher levels of stress and anxiety (from 24/7 work demands), and more diverse and sugar-rich diets to mention a few new challenges to the traditional ways to enhance health promotion.

Globalisation also affects inequality between and within countries (Becker et al., 2005). It gives rise for instance to new demands for healthcare services such as mental health treatments, which are still in the infant stages of development in many low- and middle-income countries. The latter can, in part, be attributed to a differential introduction of new health technologies and more generally improvements of standards of living, especially in the Western world evidence already indicates a significant rise in mortality among middle-aged Americans from 1993 to 2013, comparable to the trend of AIDS deaths until 2015 (Case and Deaton, 2015). However, and on the other hand, globalisation can influence poverty reduction around the world, which again feeds back in terms of higher health returns.

Global interdependence goes hand in hand with the proliferation of stakeholders that react to new global needs, which makes institutional design a more complex endeavour, but allows for tackling sources of specific health inequalities if collective action is steered accordingly. Certainly, epidemics predate the current globalisation eras as 'plague panics' of the nineteenth century (Chadavarkar, 1992); however, the threads to today's health security (e.g. global pandemics, HIV, malaria) give rise to new challenges in the governance of health systems. In addition, they bring the issue of collective action management to centre stage, as country health authorities rely more on the assistance of international organisations such as the WHO.

Finally, whilst new treatments are available, their consumption is concentrated in a small number of countries. Some evidence suggests that the richest quintile of the world population accounts for roughly 90 per cent of global healthcare spending (Benatar, 2002). This evidence is suggestive of a new rise of inequalities in access to health-care which, in part, reflects the stage of economic development countries are exposed to.

The Displacement of Global Health Investments

International cooperation in matters of public health attempts to address important global challenges, such as ensuring the diffusion of information, prevention practices and access to treatments, all of which can be regarded as 'global public goods' insofar as they require some collective action at an international level (Smith et al., 2003). However, rather than enhancing public sector cooperation, many lower-income countries, such as India and some countries in Africa, respond by expanding private or quasi-private institutions such as non-governmental organisations. This reflects, in part, the weakness of state institutions, and the limited capacity of these states to raise sufficient funds to organise a public health system. To overcome such limitations, many of those countries rely on foreign aid, but only for a selective set of conditions for which global collective action has managed to attract funds (e.g. HIV/AIDS), whilst other areas have remained neglected.

Health and population advocates in the developing world have expressed concerns that the high level of donor attention to HIV/AIDS is displacing funding for their own concerns (Shiffman, 2007). HIV/AIDS is rapidly growing as a share of total foreign aid as it receives a top priority in US funding whilst we observe a concurrent global stagnation of aid overall (Shiffman, 2007). Furthermore, the paradox here is that the level of HIV/AIDS foreign donations in several sub-Saharan African countries are such that they compare in magnitude to their entire national health budgets (Shiffman, 2007). On the other hand, aggregate donor funding for health and population quadrupled between 1992 and 2005, allowing for funding growth for some health issues even as HIV/AIDS acquired an increasingly prominent place in donor health agendas.

GLOBAL PUBLIC HEALTH NEEDS

Pandemics

Some healthcare treatments are global public goods, since they prevent the spreading of pandemics. Healthcare needs are in part communicated as a result of personal contact between different areas of the world. Many of the threats to global health, such as malaria or tuberculosis, pre-existed the development of modern medicine. But others, prominently the sub-Saharan AIDS pandemics in the 1990s, occurred after the international epidemiological transition promoted by the WHO through the spread of modern scientific-based approaches to eradicate communicable disease. Globalisation added to these threats a pandemic of chronic diseases that result from the extension of a 'global lifestyle' in terms of eating and smoking habits, which are related to the spread of information across the world. Non-communicable diseases include, for instance, cancer and respiratory diseases (e.g. Beaglehole et al., 2011). Mobility of individuals increases both the probability and the expense of these pandemics, which are estimated to cost up to 1 per cent of global GDP (Osewe, 2017).

For example, influenza epidemics account for around 10 per cent of sickness-related absence from work in Europe (Szucs et al., 2006). The latter is driven by costs to the health systems of such shocks, alongside effects on employment and productivity and wider social consequences such as, in more extreme cases, school closures and limits to mobility and consumption. The main beneficiaries of these pandemics are pharmaceutical companies producing vaccines, antibiotics and similar products. The collective action response to this challenge has resulted in a closer cooperation between the WHO and national public health agencies. However, the weakness of governance has become ever more salient. Today, it is almost impossible to mitigate the threat of an epidemic when some major country decides to opt out from multilateral regulatory agreements (e.g. China during the SARS epidemic). The latter illustrates, the failure of collective action at a global level.

To date, limited collective action has led to a weak global governance and, hence, to an inefficient allocation of public health responsibilities at the nation-state levels, irrespective of their size. The examples of the Ebola and Zika viruses illustrate the limits of national actions in guaranteeing health security, and stand out as a reminder of the world benefits of further collective action and cooperation. In a scenario of limited global governance and coordination, countries free-ride on others and rationally choose to underinvest in essential surveillance, emergency and diagnostic services which are at the core of an efficient identification and response to such outbreaks. Typically, lower-income countries have weaker capacity to respond to the need for pandemic surveillance (e.g. the outbreaks of H5N1 avian flu and A/H1N1 pandemic flu, for which vaccines and drugs were available mainly in higher-income countries), and as a result they are more likely to suffer from the consequences of limited global coordination, institutional weaknesses and restricted state capacity.

An institutional response to such needs include addressing the chronic underfunding problem by setting up a 'global insurance fund' that would protect against the continued threat of emerging infectious diseases (Berry et al., 2018). However, pooling resources to fund a globally beneficial endeavour will not spontaneously emerge, and requires overcoming present gridlock. Similarly, international treaties that reduce the national sovereignty of major international stakeholders are unlikely to take place unless major incentives are in place. Even when they are in place, enforcement is weak, and penalties mainly refer to a system of sanctions, which large countries easily overcome. Finally, even when regulation exists, often measuring compliance with international treaties is subject to loopholes, and country standards might differ.

Essential Medicines

In a similar fashion to the pandemics example, access to medical innovations is a key health input to treat numerous life-threatening conditions. However, access to such technologies is, on many occasions, limited by several market barriers, with property rights at the core. Access to medicines is still a major issue to solve in many health systems and is often regarded as part of a health security target. Multilateral trade agreements such as the Trade-Related Aspects of Intellectual Property Rights (TRIPS) are of direct concern to health information professionals. TRIPS set the minimum standards of protection for intellectual property rights, but unless compulsory (or voluntary) licences are issued, countries need to honour patent rights and cannot make necessary health technologies available to the entire population. Although patents are intended to strengthen incentives to create new knowledge, there are concerns as to the desirability of limiting and, specifically, delaying access to knowledge that is regarded as a global public good. It is still unclear whether the detrimental public health effects of barriers to the extension of medical technologies exceed the welfare effects of limiting incentives to innovation. We come back to this point in Chapter 10.

According to the World Health Survey, up to 9.5 per cent of the total household spending of poorer households in low- and middle-income countries is spent on medicines, compared to 3–5 per cent in high-income countries. This is because access to medicines in lower-income countries is significantly limited by relative high price and insurance barriers. As a way to ease the access to such technologies, the WHO developed a list of 'essential medicines' in 1977, which mainly refers to off-patent, low-priced generic medicines to treat or prevent common acute conditions. The Sustainable Development Goal 3.8 specifically mentions the importance of 'access to safe, effective, quality and affordable essential medicines and vaccines for all'; however, such a right needs to be balanced out with incentives for innovation. TRIPS oblige all member countries to provide patents for all technologies, including pharmaceuticals, with a minimum duration of twenty years. It also includes a range of flexibilities that provide governments with options that allow for the protection of public health, including access to affordable medicines (Wirtz et al., 2017).

Cooperative solutions to the question of access to medicines entail the mobilisation of stakeholders, including the pharmaceutical industry, to make specific proposals that both address needs of health securing (avoiding fake copies) and reduce barriers to access to quality-assured affordable medicines. In this spirit, the 2008 Human Rights Guidelines for Pharmaceutical Companies in Relation to Access to Medicines and the 2011 UN Guiding Principles on Business and Human Rights attempt to balance the two conflicting principles of guaranteeing public health on the one hand and innovation goals of medicines on the other hand (Wirtz et al., 2017). Among the several proposals lies the identification of 'new essential medicines', the price of which can then be delinked from development costs, and hence made available at affordable prices by means of non-exclusive licensing agreements. However, one of the potential risks is that needs that are particular to low-income countries become neglected in a market-based model, which calls for government intervention both at the national and international level. One of the proposals is an 'Essential Medicines Patent Pool' to provide the R&D to continue to cater to the needs of lower-income countries, promoting local production to encourage affordable generic access. For instance, Mozambique received support from the government of Brazil to promote domestic low-cost antiretrovirals (Wirtz et al., 2017).

Disease Prevention

The failure of collective action to address the unexpected effects of globalisation has led to major epidemics. Costa-Font and Mas (2016) found that although globalisation as a whole tends to be associated with an increase in obesity rates, more specifically changes in 'social' lifestyles related to globalisation (e.g. changes in information flows) are the main drivers of such effects. Overweight, obesity and diet-related non-communicable diseases (NCDs) have greatly increased in low- and middle-income countries, in which more than 80 per cent of deaths from NCDs worldwide already take place. These emerging NCDs coexist with undernutrition, demonstrating the so-called double burden of malnutrition (Wahlqvist, 2006). The sudden globalisation in Eastern Europe was a shock that had long-term consequences. For instance, between 1989 and 1994, life expectancy in Russia declined by more than 6.7 years in men and by 3.4 years in women due to the effects of the transition process (Shkolnikov, 1997). Trade openness has brought an increasing expansion of tobacco consumption, which today is mostly a habit of poor people in both low- and high-income countries. This explains why the tobacco lobbyists have been an active advocate for further trade liberalisation (Woodward et al., 2002). Deaths attributable to tobacco between 2002 and 2030 are set to decline by 9 per cent in high-income countries, but to double from 3.4 million to 6.8 million in low- and middle-income countries (Mathers and Loncar, 2006). This points to the need to strengthen global health governance.

GLOBAL HEALTH GOVERNANCE

The most important limits of collective action at the global level, include a weak national regulation (Rosecrance, 1999), and national governments prioritisation of economic development over public health goals. Examples include the default position of governments to encourage mobility of goods and services even after the outbreak of an epidemic. Similarly, patient protection, which is typically enacted to encourage innovation, is traded off against public health goals, which has led some countries to undertake compulsory licensing of existing technologies. Indeed, the unavailability of patented health technologies hampers population health in low-income countries and, more generally, the financing of drugs through patents leads to limited investment in orphan treatments and technologies that benefit primarily the populations of low-income countries. The emergence of health crises (e.g. need for antiretrovirals) when companies do not voluntarily license the production of technologies, has led to the issuing of compulsory licences for such drugs.

An additional potential response to the problem of collective action includes the identification of 'spaces of global governance' where countries cooperate to confront global stakeholders. That is, the creation of 'clubs' of nations which institutionalise the international cooperation of states as non-state stakeholders. An example of the latter is the role of the WHO in setting Millennium Development Goals (MDGs), which implicitly have global health governance through a Pandemic Preparedness Framework, or the global Code of Practice on the International Recruitment of Health Personnel. Similarly, the UN Security Council has adopted resolutions on HIV/AIDS and Ebola, given that such conditions have been commonly portrayed as a risk to peace and security.

Donor states increase development assistance for health through bilateral aid alongside the Global Fund. This global aid bypasses traditional institutions, such as the WHO or the World Bank, alongside initiatives by the G8, and extensive NGO involvement. New and unprecedented institutional arrangements have arisen to address anti-smoking campaigns such as the 2003 Framework Convention on Tobacco Control (FCTC), the first time the WHO adopted a treaty under Article 19 of the WHO Constitution. However, one of the endemic problems of such organisations is that developing countries have limited effective power in them due to their limited financial capabilities and human resource shortages (Deaton, 2004). Hence, higher-income countries hold a disproportionately elevated influence.

Low-income countries more likely on average, to prioritise economic development over public health goals. A paradigmatic example can be found in many African countries. Although after independence, Africa exhibited significant advances in healthcare (e.g. the expansion of health insurance coverage, large-scale campaigns against specific infectious diseases, health investments and training of health workers), globalisation has reverted part of such accomplishments with the emergence of new infectious diseases and the resurgence of eradicated ones (Iliffe, 1995). Economic stagnation only worsened the situation (in many countries of West Asia and sub-Saharan Africa, per capita income levels have fallen below those of the 1970s), resulting in an expansion of a significant growth of global external debt, notable cuts in healthcare services and the consequent weakening of the state, the erosion of democracy and the emergence of ethnic grievances (Fidler, 2010).

Economic stagnation coincided with the 1995 General Agreement on Trade in Services (GATS), which required governments to open national health services to international commercial suppliers of health services, which more generally gave rise to the privatisation of healthcare services in many countries. Some argue that, given that poorer populations are more likely to use public healthcare, privatisation is partially responsible for access to only limited-to-basic healthcare in such groups (Deaton, 2004). Government stewardship is needed to avoid regulatory capture by vested interests and corruption, as we discuss in Part III of the book.

Healthcare stakeholders, unlike many national states, have reacted to the demands of globalisation by developing 'international networks' of manufacturers of originators. Such stakeholders play a role as veto players of major reforms that change the existing status quo in the way healthcare markets operate across the world. Lobbying has become an integral and costly part of the diffusion efforts of manufacturers worldwide, which makes global collective action even more complex, and difficult for self-interested stakeholders.

PROFESSIONAL AND PATIENT MOBILITY

International Professional Mobility

One of the immediate effects of increasingly interdependent economies is the mobility of health professionals to those countries offering better standards of living. However, professional mobility comes at the cost of free-riding on the training investment of other countries and their needs. In 2011, the WHO estimated that fifty-four countries were still facing critical shortages of medical staff. India and the Philippines account for the largest shares of migrant doctors and nurses working in Organisation for Economic Co-operation and Development (OECD) countries. The WHO estimated that in 2006, there was a shortage of 4.3 million health personnel across the world, especially affecting low-income countries, with fifty-seven nations in a state of critical shortage (WHO, 2010). The share of foreign-born doctors increased in most countries between 2000/1 and 2010/11, rising from 19.5 per cent to 22 per cent across twenty-three OECD countries (Buchan et al., 2017). For instance, after 2004 Germany and the UK exhibited a notable growth in the number of Polish doctors (Buchan et al., 2017). Although the USA receives the highest number of migrant doctors and nurses in absolute terms, the steepest rises in foreign-born doctors, as shown in Table 3.2, have been recorded in Germany and the UK alongside Australia, Ireland, New Zealand and Switzerland. In contrast, other countries that are mainly exporters of doctors, such as Poland or Mexico, envisage little to no change. Although globally there are more than enough health workers to meet the needs of the world population, there are shortages in some countries, especially low- and middle-income countries. Importantly, future jobs are not necessarily created in the areas where there is the most need. Buchan et al. (2017) show that whilst shortages decline in almost all countries, they are expected to rise by a magnitude of 45 per cent in a decade in Africa.

International Patient Mobility

Alongside labour mobility, globalisation steer patient mobility too. International health mobility refers to travels from one country to another for the purpose of obtaining medical treatment. Traditionally, people travel from less-developed countries, to major medical centres in highly developed countries for medical treatments that are unavailable in their own communities (Horowitz et al., 2007). Examples of the latter include Hospital 'Bambino Gesù' initiatives in Rome treating African children for very complex interventions (such as separating conjoined twins). However, 'medical tourism' is likely to expand due to the development of global standards of quality, providers' accreditation (Segouin et al., 2005), and more generally specific needs associated with the tourism industry (e.g. Qatar is investing in hospitals in Sardinia). However, nowadays the direction of travel is

Table 3.2 *Share (%) of foreign doctors and nurses in selected OECD countries*

Years	Doctors		Nurses	
	2000	2010	2000	2010
Australia	43	53	25	33
Austria	15	17	14	15
Belgium	12	25	7	17
Canada	35	35	17	22
Denmark	11	19	4	10
Finland	4	8	1	2
France	17	19	5	6
Germany	11	16	10	14
Hungary	11	13	3	2
Ireland	36	47	14	27
Mexico	1	1	0.2	0.2
Netherlands	17	15	7	10
New Zealand	47	54	23	35
Poland	3	3	0.4	0.2
Portugal	20	16	14	9
Spain	7	10	3	6
Sweden	23	30	9	14
Switzerland	28	42	29	33
UK	34	35	15	22
USA	25	26	12	15
OECD	20	24	11	14

Source: OECD Health Statistics 2015 (www.oecd.org/health)

often both ways. The exclusion of public insurance coverage of certain procedures, prominently dental healthcare, becomes an incentive for mobility, in Italy for instance, towards less expensive bordering countries like Slovenia or close countries like Croatia. Small countries such as Kuwait find is cheaper to reimburse healthcare abroad that to invest of new health care facilities.

DOES THE PATIENT CITIZEN GAIN FROM GLOBALISATION?

Given the absence of a strong global governance for healthcare, a question that emerges is: does the patient citizen (PC) gain from globalisation? Globalisation facilitates the transmission of health knowledge and the diffusion of health technology, mainly by lowering the costs of trade and exchange. This includes information and communication technologies, pharmaceuticals and medical devices that allow for improvements in prevention and care (e.g. intensive care units, screening equipment, etc.). However, the enaction of costly technologies, which encompasses new training needs, creates a 'technological divide'. For instance, in the case of tele-diagnostics and the use of the Internet for medical purposes is not equally used by different population groups, which can potentially give rise to a two-tier system.

Similarly, globalisation has also affected the international distribution of income across countries. The idea is that new health technologies are diffused and adopted first in rich countries, which creates a technological divide sharpening the health gradient, in other words the widely observed positive correlation between health status and income. Then, to moderate the health gradient, diffusion and access to innovation in poor countries has to be encouraged and this might be one of the policy priorities of global health in the years to come. This is more important between than within countries, and patient mobility would be more likely to solve differences within countries whilst mobility is lower between countries.

By reducing transaction costs for the trade of goods and services, and increasing interdependence, globalisation inevitably gives rise to some level of competition between health systems to attract talent and technology at the lowest possible cost. As in the inter-jurisdictional interactions discussed in Chapter 2, it is possible to observe either a race to the top ('a race of quality improvement') or a race to the bottom ('a race of cutting costs'). One reaction to competition is to make health systems more differentiated and specific (e.g. special training and accreditation systems), which can largely limit the extent of mobility possible. However, globalisation allows for the diffusion of international best practices, which might close the gaps between systems, except when the best practices require some investment, in which case they may exacerbate cross-country differences.

An alternative explanation is the 'compensation thesis' (Cameron, 1978), which states that by extending healthcare coverage and, more generally, compensating losers of globalisation, governments square the support necessary for re-election and keep globalisation running. This explains why 89 per cent of all global healthcare activity takes place in 16 per cent of the world's population (Benatar, 2002). Whilst sub-Saharan Africa spends less than 2 per cent of its GDP on healthcare, the USA spends 17 per cent, which is not the result of differences in preferences, but in degrees of economic development. At a lower level of development maximising health is more important than its distribution (Costa-Font et al., 2018). More generally, the benefits of globalisation on health tend to be concentrated in high- and middle-income countries, a feature that is exemplified by the overwhelming concentration of global health crises in Africa and lower-income countries.

Globalisation empowers the role of multinational corporations and international organisations. Multinational corporations can use the threat of capital flight to pressure governments into pursuing certain reforms that benefit their industry. Medical industries provide a large number of jobs that would be at risk after relocation. Hence, globalisation gives rise to a new form of global governance. Liberalisation and deregulation of health-related industries have taken place around the world in different formats. Some of the more extreme, such as the deregulation of drug authorisation in Peru, led to a significant rise in drug prices as patients and providers shifted their trust towards medicines delivered by international companies rather than local ones (Costa-Font, 2016).

Similarly, the role of the private sector differs across countries, and globalisation of trade helps to expand its influence. However, not all states have enough state capacity to monitor the increasing 'privatisation' of new healthcare programmes, meaning that these are programmes which tend to benefit a smaller share of the population than in the past. Similarly, the expansion of globalisation coincides with an expansion of worldwide inequality, which can give rise to a negative effect on health (Deaton, 2004). Inequality can make some specific countries and populations more vulnerable to the health risks.

The imbalances of globalisation are related to historical legacies such as colonialism, weaker rule of law, limited access to information and frail democracy, and, more generally, weaker economic development. These cross-country differences illustrate the unbalanced nature of power, where a small set of countries hold an overwhelming influence in future access to healthcare and healthy inputs over the rest of the population. Finally, globalisation gives rise to some form of 'global communication', and hence can open the door to further ideological dominance of advocacy groups and vested interests calling for different, and often opposing, goals such as openness or closing up of society and the economy, cosmopolitanism or localism, etc. We come back to the role of ideas and ideology in Chapter 7.

SUMMARY

We have argued that the attainment of global public health goals requires overcoming 'global collective inaction'. When global healthcare governance is limited to the nation state, countries exhibit considerable incentives to free-ride on actions of others. The governance of health systems has, in turn, become more complex as a result of a globalisation process that brings new stakeholders into the fore, and new, well-organised demands that have steered collective action, such as with HIV/AIDS, have displaced other sources of development aid.

Healthcare is increasingly standardised with the diffusion of new technologies previously unavailable, but even standardised treatment brings new risks in the form of pandemics. The development of global pandemics call for coordinated actions, and ultimately for the strengthening of global governance. In recent years we have seen the proliferation of several types of institutional responses to the need of global governance, consistently suggesting the view that institutions emerge as a result of the need to solve coordination problems.

The transition to globalisation has entailed the diffusion of Western lifestyles, and some of these new lifestyles are the result of the adoption of social norms that pre-existing ones governing health-related behavior. As a result, estimates suggest an expansion of health inequalities on a global scale, which is reflected in the rise in obesity rates in low- and middle-income countries (Mexico, Brazil), alongside the shift of tobacco consumption towards low- and middle-income countries. The increasing standardisation of health technologies means that patients are willing to travel to attain either better access, better quality or a lower cost of care. On the other hand, healthcare professional mobility means that, increasingly, many developed countries exhibit a significant share of foreign professionals which might give rise to shortages in many sending countries that cannot retain them.

PART III   Political Institutions and Health

4 Constitutional Health System Design

CONSTITUTIONS AND HEALTHCARE

Health systems are part of a wider macro-level design establishing the principles and 'rules of the game' a society should be guided by. Such choices include principles that constrain policy choices to respect for human and economics rights. Such choices, in turn, influence the behaviour and expectations of the patient citizen (PC). The morphology of a health system is determined by so-called first-level choices,[1] representaives of the PC make, in constitutional commissions and in Parliament. Among those first-level choices, one should highlight the delineation of how political power is shared horizontally (between the executive, judiciary and legislative branches of government). In making such first-level choices, countries are deemed to decide whether healthcare is regulated as a human right. Specifically, the right to the highest attainable standard of health which was included in the Constitution of the World Health Organization (WHO) back in 1946. However, the way this right to health is implemented and prioritised differs across countries, and we still know little about how constitutions, which define the basic institutions of a country, influence healthcare activity alongside the PC's access to health services.

This chapter focuses on how the consideration of the constitutional rights to healthcare influence healthcare activity and outcomes. The prioritisation of some constitutional rights (e.g. universal access to healthcare) might be at the expense of other health system objectives (Matsuura, 2014). The rest of the chapter examines how the articulation of political power is horizontally shared, and whether a

[1] That is, choices about the institutions of a country, as opposed to second-order-level choices that are made within the frame of such institutions (Wildavsky, 1987).

country adopts a parliamentary as opposed to presidential typology of state organisation, the type of electoral system to aggregate individuals' public preferences for healthcare policies, all influence the health system dynamics, and healthcare spending. We then go on to argue that such constitutional provisions influence how health services are financed and organised.

Next, we illustrate how the constitutional prerogatives influence health system performance, especially when different stakeholders in a country disagree on the direction of reform the health system should take. Earlier, we pointed out that constitutional conflicts around how best to design the health system are frequent in Western societies, illustrated by the recent constitutional legal appeal of the Affordable Care Act (ACA) in the United States. Similarly, as described in Chapter 2, in countries such as Germany, Canada, Spain or Italy, constitutional conflicts routinely emerge between the regional/state and the central/federal governments, both of whom compete for the execution of major healthcare responsibilities (Costa-Font and Rico, 2006a; Montolio and Turati, 2017). This is because most constitutions are 'incomplete contracts' which cannot foresee *ex ante* all possible future conflicts. Hence, they tend to define a few principles that need interpretation.

THE CONSTITUTIONAL RIGHT TO HEALTH

An important way to promote health, and constrain future government attempts to downplay the primacy of health, is the specific mention of the right to health in national and state constitutions. In addition to constraining government action directly, it allows the PC to appeal to the judiciary when governments fail to align their priorities with constitutional prerogatives (Mulumba et al., 2010). Indeed, when such a right is recognised, the courts can play an active role in enforcing it when the government fails to honour it. This is especially important when countries have not yet achieved universal health coverage. An example of healthcare access regulation in the United States is the Emergency Medical Treatment and Active

Labor Act (EMTALA) which ensures Americans' access to emergency medical care. Another example refers to anti-discrimination legislation passed after the civil rights movements in the USA, protecting the rights of ethnic minorities as well as the rights of disabled and undocumented migrants (Matsuura, 2014). However, the constitutional inclusion of the right to healthcare does not automatically entail that all barriers to the access of healthcare are lifted. This is because regulations do not automatically give rise to specific policies to reduce such barriers (e.g. waiting times, congestion, cost-sharing, etc.). An example of the latter can be found in the actual implementation of EMTALA, which has no associated funding and can give rise to hospital congestion in admitting emergency patients.

The right to health has been, historically, a relatively recent incorporation in modern countries' legislations. Indeed, it was not included as part of international treaties, nor in national constitutions until the second half of the twentieth century. Paradoxically, the country pioneering the introduction of such a right was the USSR in its 1936 Constitution, which defined, for the first time, the right of access to healthcare. After the Second World War the right to health was sanctioned in the constitutions of several democratic countries. This began in Italy in 1947, and was followed by the provision of an 'adequate' level of medical care in the Universal Declaration of Human Rights (UDHR). Subsequently, the right to health was adopted by the fifty-six members of the United Nations in 1948, followed by the Declaration of Alma Ata in 1978, which elaborated on the meaning of such a right (Matsuura, 2014). Although some constitutions do not include this right, the right to healthcare has been activated by constitutional courts as an extension of other rights. An example of the latter is the interpretation of the Supreme Court of India, which refers to the right to health as an extension to the protection of life and personal liberty (WHO, 2011).

Healthcare services are not explicitly mentioned in the founding treaties of the current European Union, with the exception of Article 3 of the Treaty of the European Commission (TEC), that states that the European Community shall contribute to a 'high level of health protection'. However, over time the EU has extended its remit to act in a number of areas such as international and public health and blood donation, alongside products and services affected by the single market such as medicines and medical devices. Since the 1990s the European Court of Justice (ECJ) has responded with a row of cases by granting foreign workers the right to access the guest state's healthcare system (Anderson, 2015). More generally, the ECJ has played an active role in defining the jurisdiction of European institutions, especially in healthcare, although social policy is typically a responsibility allocated to European Union member states (Greer, 2008). This has taken place, despite the European Union being criticised for its 'constitutional asymmetry', privileging the 'economic sphere' over the 'social sphere' (Scharpf, 2002), the European Council has more recently been active in setting out its common principles to guide EU healthcare systems in 2006, which include the values of universality, access to good-quality care, equity and solidarity (European Commission, 2007). More recently, the patient mobility directive (2011/24/EU) sets out clearly the right of cross-border healthcare in accordance with the rulings of the ECJ (Greer, 2008). It grants patients free movement in the EU and additionally the right to receive non-hospital care in another member state. Hence, even at the European level, healthcare rights are increasingly being acknowledged both at the country and, especially, at the Europe-wide level.

Yet, does the inclusion of the 'right to healthcare' make a difference? The evidence on this matter is still scarce, but some already shows that infant and under-five mortality rates decreased significantly after countries introduced a right to health provision in their national constitutions (Matsuura, 2013). These results are consistent with previous evidence that finds that in the United States, state constitutions with stronger constitutional commitment to health exhibited lower infant mortality rates (Matsuura, 2012). That is, the constitutional recognition of the right to healthcare can open up the institutional mechanisms that call for more active governmental activity in expanding social protection in healthcare.

CONSTITUTIONAL TRADE-OFFS AND VETO POINTS

Health system design, in theory, is the reflection of beliefs about the rights to well-being while in practice they readily coexist with fundamental socio-political inequalities operating within a country (WHO, 2008). Early economic analysis of health system designs (Breyer, 1995) already revealed the importance of political determinants, especially in social insurance systems. This is because under tight budget constraints, an expansion of healthcare expenditures frequently occurs at the expense of other investments in infrastructures and other public outlays. That is, governments are forced to trade off health policy goals against other goals. Similarly, the role of markets in the provision of healthcare can be both inhibited or encouraged in the constitutional provisions and its companion legislation. The same applies to the health systems' role in curbing health inequality, which is included as an implicit or explicit goal of the health systems in most constitutions of European countries, but it not always the case that they manage to reduce health inequality.

The constitutional design of political institutions shapes the agenda-setting of healthcare reforms. For instance, parliamentary democracies tend to assign to the parliament an active role in initiating legislation, hence one would expect more health care reform initiatives to go through (though not necessarily to be more successful). This is because parliamentary systems exert lesser control by the executive over the reform agenda, than in presidential systems. Political competition and political incentives influence both reform sources and public expenditure expansion, but both competition and incentives are conditional to the constitutional arrangements of a country. To understand this, it is useful to distinguish political decision-making in two main stages (also known as two level games): (i) the first is the constitutional stage, which defines the main/meta rules of the game within which the (ii) policy process or policymaking is then developed and applied, for example through following the will of the median voter. There is clearly a balance between the two stages (Buchanan, 1975b); however, the design of constitutions often is blurred in attributing authority. In the latter case, blurred constitutional provisions tend to provide a more active role to the constitutional courts (e.g. the Supreme Court in the USA or the ECJ in Europe) in interpreting the constitution or the treaties, or aspects around the 'right to healthcare'.

It is possible to argue that there is also an inherent conflict and/ or tension, where a rigid constitution might be seen as a way to maintain the status quo and the privileges of the elites, while on the other hand the ordinary policy process (under flexible constitutions) might trump the constitutional limits and push polities towards the dictatorship of the majority, if not towards anarchy.

The tension between rigid and flexible constitutions is relevant in defining the institutional morphology of a health system. In cases where constitutions do not specifically refer to the right to healthcare, it still is a quasi-constitutional arrangement (Cutler and Johnson, 2004; Congleton and Bose, 2010), as it is often difficult to revert or drastically modify implemented health policies. This is because ideological views consolidate through time for the presence of veto players within the health system decision-making process. But constitutions can influence health systems in a more nuanced way as they also define in detail other characteristics of the government. One way constitutions influence health systems is by defining how power is vertically allocated, namely defining the prerogatives of central and subcentral governments (which has already been discussed in Chapter 2), but simultaneously, how it is allocated horizontally, namely the explicit role of the executive and legislative powers in defining health reform, as well as the role of the judiciary in its implementation. Similarly, constitutions legislate on how preferences over healthcare reforms are aggregated, and more specifically, they tend to delimit the electoral system (proportional or majoritarian), that lead to the selection of the representative of the PC. Persson and Tabellini (2004) illustrate the importance of the constitutional allocation of power and, more specifically, whether the policy initiative (selection process) lies in the hands of the executive (presidential) or the legislative (parliamentary) play an important role in policymaking and the budget size of the government, including the public health system. For instance, countries that aggregate preferences via proportional representation are likely to produce higher levels of public expenditure (Persson and Tabellini, 2004).

If we proceed with the standard tripartition together with the executive and legislative powers, there is also the judiciary. But literature on the judiciary has not addressed the healthcare sector as far as we know, maybe with the exception of new developments that are still ongoing with regards to the constitutionality of Obamacare. However, it can be said, paralleling the literature on the judiciary, that committees that evaluate the quality and effectiveness of, for example, a new health technology (Food and Drug Administration, or FDA), are acting as judges or committees of judges. This gives rise to a possible defensive and asymmetric approval process, where taking the risk of passing a harmful drug is considered socially and politically more costly than rejecting drugs which would have been beneficial for the target population. There might well be political factors that give more weight to one type of error over another, with the consequence of creating a more risk-taking or risk-avoiding committee.

Another important aspect we address here is the articulation of power through the distribution of veto players (Tsebelis, 1995, 2002). This power is in the capacity of stopping the new policy proposals. Constitutions often foresee prerogatives to aim at granting stability that provide some bodies veto power or limit significantly the capacity to introduce policy proposals. This explains why some proposals such as the Clinton healthcare reform in the 1990s and some parts of Obamacare were not included in the final draft of the legislation (such as the CLASS Act). More generally, in every country there have been reform proposals that have been paralysed or buried due to a veto of some majority party in one of the parliamentary chambers.

Finally, health decision-making is also affected and shaped on the basis of the independence that healthcare institutions enjoy with respect to the other branches of government. Public agencies that are dependent upon government funds for support render decisions as being subject to political influence. Similarly, the decentralisation of healthcare responsibilities in many federal and quasi-federal countries is regulated by a framework law. However, it is often the case that the interpretation of such legislation by judges and constitutional courts can be heterogeneous, and deviate over time, which suggests that even judges are not totally independent from more general political problems.

THE ALLOCATION OF POWER-SHARING

Horizontal Power-Sharing

Most world states are organised to separate powers in the form of judicial, executive and legislative, the latter often articulated in two separate chambers of decision-making (bicameral). Elster (1994) argues that power separation plays a role in protecting citizens against time inconsistency, as it acts as a pre-commitment device. These structures can be reproduced both at the supra-state (e.g. European Commission, European Parliament and Court of Justice) and the sub-state level (e.g. regional parliaments, executives). This power separation can play an important role in making sure that government's regulation in healthcare is accountable to its citizens by ensuring the so-called mutual guardship of citizens' needs, and especially by protecting them against corruption.

Checks and Balances

The constitutional design of the health system influences the institutional dynamics of the processes of healthcare reform. This applies indirectly even when the health system is an independent organisation, such as a social insurance fund, or directly when ministers and secretaries of state for health are politically accountable to parliament. Typically, parliamentary discussions by opposition parties will take advantage of specific health crises to increase the salience of health issues. However, the latter depends on the specific governmental system in place. Health systems in a strong presidential setting are less likely to exhibit leadership in issuing legislative proposals. In contrast, those systems where the parliament plays a key role in legislative initiations face a larger number of vetoes. The example of the ACA in the USA is illustrative of the significant amendments that a law must undergo before it can attract a pronounced majority in both Congress and Senate. Although originally the reform was conceived by a form of social insurance, it was progressively amended to allow for insurance choice. In such settings, logrolling and government negotiation to satisfy the interests of different stakeholders were required for the legislation to pass.

ELECTORAL COMPETITION

The Electoral System

In choosing an electoral system, a common trade-off that the literature highlights is between *accountability and representation* (Persson and Tabellini, 2004). For instance, in elections guided by plurality (or majority rule), small swings in some key states might give rise to significant differences in parliamentary majorities. These might imply stronger accountability and smaller incentives to engage in corruption, as we will discuss in Chapter 8. The downside is that the system will implement the healthcare reforms supported by a small share of pivotal voters that 'make a difference' for the electoral results. In contrast, electoral systems organised around principles of proportional representation are more likely to require a wider base of support and give rise to coalition governments. Coalition governments have different spending preferences than single-party governments, and are more likely to spend more on healthcare as there might be competing views to satisfy. Persson and Tabellini (2003) find salient welfare-state spending expansions in election and post-election years in proportional representation systems, but not in plurality systems.

Competition between parties is arguably desirable, insofar as it gives rise to legislation that pleases voters at large (Persson and

Tabellini, 2004). An increase in party competition can contribute to an upward movement in health expenditure expansion if the financing is less transparent and the costs are diffused across the population. The example of the ACA shows that, although the subsidy was put forward by the federal government, some of the costs of the health insurance mandate fell into the hands of small and mid-sized businesses for whom the provision of insurance entails a significant cost. However, the ACA was overall perceived as popular among the electorate, so expanding health insurance in the USA was perceived as bringing electoral returns. In contrast, in India, Saez and Sinha (2010) show evidence that governments reduce expenditure on health around the time of elections. This evidence suggests incumbents' incentives to invest in health are low and sensitive to the electoral cycle. Incumbents have tended to opportunistically increase the growth of public health expenditures in election years in Organisation for Economic Co-operation and Development (OECD) countries during the 1971–2004 period (Potrafke, 2010).

For Figure 4.1, we merged World Development Indicators data on total and public health spending with the Proportional Representation (PR) variable from the Database of Political Institutions (DPI; 2017). The same sources were used for Figures 4.2 and 4.3. We show

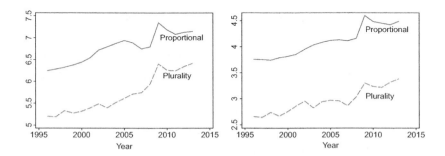

FIGURE 4.1 Total (right) and public (left) health spending and the electoral system: proportional representation versus plurality

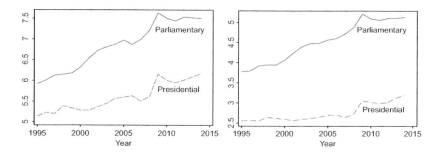

FIGURE 4.2 Total (right) and public (left) health spending and the political system: presidential versus parliamentary

the time series for the 1995–2014 period according to the electoral system. Figure 4.1 shows that proportional systems tend both to display higher and steeper total and public health spending as a percentage of GDP.

Figure 4.2 instead reveals a similar trend of total and public health spending as a percentage of GDP, estimated using data from the DPI (2017). Originally, this variable was multi-categorical with a value equal to 2 for parliamentary systems, 1 for political systems with an assembly-elected president and 0 for purely presidential ones. We then modified to classify a parliamentary system for original values equal to 2 or 1, and equal to 0 if the SYSTEM variable was equal to 0. Consistently with Persson and Tabellini (2003), we find that parliamentary systems spend more in terms of GDP both in total and public health spending.

Electoral Incentives and Healthcare Reform

Healthcare reform proposals, however, require majorities in the electorate to succeed. Re-election incentives have been shown to affect economic policy choices (Besley and Case, 1993), and the distribution of voter incomes. The expected change in voter support from varying levels of public provision correlates the allocation of government expenditure (Tridimas, 2001). Pensioners and chronic patients and their families, who rely on benefits from the public health system are not likely to vote for reform. The ACA experience illustrates how policy makers seek to put forward reforms that satisfy the preferences of certain groups at the expense of others, and ultimately policy decisions face the need to square a trade-off between efficiency or equity perspectives. This applies to specific programmes such as the cancer screening of certain conditions, or the introduction of a new health treatment, irrespective of their value. In the context of pharmaceutical reforms, Reich (1995) finds that strong and narrow political coalition improve the capacity of political leaders to resist the pressures of concentrated economic costs (both inside and outside national boundaries). Finally, health policies need some electoral legitimacy to secure support from wider electoral coalition especially, if they entail a redistribution component. That said, policies directed at the poor may receive less popular support because the median voter does not perceive any personal or family need for such services.

Some voters will not be satisfied by the public healthcare system for a variety of reasons. Typically they are those with higher need for healthcare and also have larger incomes at their disposal (Epple and Romano, 1996a, 1996b). Given that healthcare is a normal good, individuals with larger incomes have greater willingness and ability to pay for healthcare, for example, either out-of-pocket or via supplemental private health insurance if this is allowed. Strategically, they might also prefer not to cross-subsidise poorer, sicker people through public spending. High-income voters may therefore prefer a lower level of public health spending, especially when they have the option of private health insurance, and this will move the median voter demand down. Evidence for this has been found in OECD countries (Tuohy et al., 2004). However, Epple and Romano (1996b) argue that if income effects are weak, low- and high-income taxpayers are not that interested in paying taxes to get healthcare unless heavily subsidised, if not free. We return to this point in Chapter 6.

VETO PLAYERS AND AGENDA-SETTING

The larger the number of parties involved in the decision-making process the more important the veto power of some of the stakeholders (Tsebelis, 1995, 2002). Presidential systems often allow the president to veto legislation. Similarly, the strength of the executive led by a presidential system as opposed to a parliamentary system confers to the latter more influence in the agenda-setting. In presidential systems, given that the executive is directly elected, it has stronger legitimacy to initiate legislation than the executives in parliamentary systems. In parliamentary regimes, in contrast, the government concentrates the main, but not all prerogatives as well as important powers of initiating legislation. Checks and balances are thus stronger under presidential governments, and government decisions cater to a wider base under parliamentary systems. Persson and Tabellini (2004) estimate that switching from a parliamentary to a presidential system would reduce public spending by 5 per cent of GDP. However, it does not look at health care spending in particular.

Figure 4.3 shows instead the association between total and public health spending as a percentage of GDP and a measure of veto power strength. To construct this variable, we use the DPI (2017) dataset. We collect information on the 'longest tenure of a veto

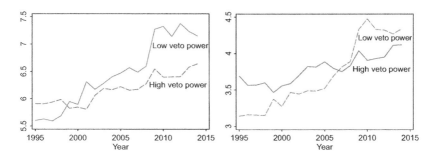

FIGURE 4.3 Total (right) and public (left) health spending and 'high' versus 'low' veto power

player', which 'measures the tenure of the veto player in a country as reported by the raw information of the Legislative and Executive Indices of Electoral Competitiveness (LIEC). We classify countries as having high and low veto power, based on the values being values above-below the median. We then document two facts. First, trends of both total and public spending are different for high and low veto countries, which is consistent with the idea that vetoing has the effect of restricting health care reform, and keeping decisions closer to the status quo. Second, we find that although high veto power countries were initially spending more than low ones, during the last two decades, countries with low veto power were able to increase their spending more than countries with high veto power. In contrast, low veto power countries surpassed, on average, spending in high veto countries, though recently there has been no clear indication if the wedge created is expanding or reducing.

SUMMARY

This chapter has examined how the constitutional design of a health system plays a role in the evolution of healthcare activity. We have argued that when a constitution defines the primacy of social rights to healthcare, it actually limits the capacity of future minority governments to restrict them, and allows the PC to invoke his/her right when violated. In other words, constitutions act as macro institution devices to ensure that government action takes place within defined limits.

We have illustrated how explicit constitutional provisions, choice of the electoral system, the type of political system and the presence of veto points can all influence healthcare activity. In all cases we show that proportional representation, parliamentary system and lower veto points tend to give rise to higher expenditures. This evidence overall indicates that the constitutional design of the health system influences its dynamics of reform and performance as well as the scrutiny and agenda-setting of executives' powers in pushing for change.

5 Democracy and the Patient Citizen

5

WHY DOES DEMOCRACY MATTER?

The organisation of health services tends to reflect the values and priorities of each population. However, as we discussed in Chapter 1, healthcare, unlike other areas of public interventions, is affected by significant information asymmetries between patients and providers (Dulleck and Kerschbamer, 2006), which influence the way the patient citizen (PC) expresses its demands for healthcare. As discussed in Chapter 4, the constitutional design of a country – including the electoral rules, the division of powers and the role of the judiciary – adds additional veto players into the health system reform process, and often extra 'checks and balances' that are not always in the interest of the PC. At the core of those institutions lie the mechanisms of accountability (to the PC) and representation (of the view of the PC). That is, a well-functioning democracy would be one where healthcare decisions are the expression of the PC's demands. Such demands are typically revealed through electoral processes (which turn heterogeneous preferences into political mandates), as we discuss later in Chapter 6. However, as a first step to understand how health policy choices are made, we discuss whether and how democratic decision-making, unlike other political collective decision-making systems, affects the health system.

This chapter provides an overview of the research linking democracy and democratic transitions to health outcomes and healthcare policymaking.[1] We examine the processes and institutions that

---

[1] More specifically, we look here at regime transitions from autocratic to democratic. In Chapter 4 we explored the relationship between *types* of democracies and health. Types of democracies have been defined as to whether democratic systems are

influence health directly, or indirectly, by affecting the access and availability of healthcare and other inputs in the health production process, such as economic prosperity (Acemoglu and Robinson, 2013). In one of the earliest empirical analyses gauging the effect of democracy on health outcomes, Besley and Kudamatsu (2006, p. 313) write: 'which aspects of policy making and human well-being are promoted by democracies is still a subject of debate'. There is, in fact, little doubt that democratisation represents an essential shift of the political system of a country, and through the rest of the chapter we will offer a review of the literature on how democratic transitions and consolidations affect health outcomes, and on the mediating mechanisms linking democracy to health. There are several potential mechanisms that can explain how democracy, and more specifically democratic institutions, affect the delivery of health services. Perhaps the most apparent way to describe it is through the agency relationship between decision makers and the PC, which hence makes the political demand for healthcare. Similarly, as we will discuss in Chapter 6, electoral processes allow self-interested parties competing for the electoral suppport of the PC (as health care tops the policy priorities in most countries) and accommodate its political healthcare demands. However, it is not uncommon that political priorities do not align with the preferences and needs of neglected population groups.

Democratic processes can influence the allocation of healthcare resources in several ways. Betancourt and Gleason (2000) find that while a higher voter turnout in a district increases the allocation of nurses to its rural areas, it does not affect the allocation of doctors. Similarly, Mobarak et al. (2011) find, using data from Brazil, that the number of public clinics and consultation rooms – the visible public goods – are positively related to voter turnout, but not to the number of doctors and nurses. Health inequalities persist in many countries despite the existence of democratic institutions, which calls for a

proportional/presidential; with electoral systems that are proportional/majoritarian; if the structure of the state and the organisation of public healthcare provision is more/less centralised or whether it depends on voters' and politicians' ideology (see Chapter 7). See, for example Altman et al. (2017) for a recent contribution.

further study of how transitions to more democratic institutions influence healthcare policies and reforms. However, before we discuss such mechanisms, we first present the empirical evidence on the effect of democracy on health. Next, we enumerate potential mechanisms explaining the evidence, and then we try to answer the following questions: What are the mediating effects of the extension of voting rights, inequality and other explanations? When does democracy fail in improving health and reducing health inequalities?

IS THERE A HEALTH DIVIDEND FROM DEMOCRACY?

What Do We Mean by Democracy?

A starting point in studying the effect of democracy on health and healthcare lies in testing whether different measures of democracy correlate with health measures. In doing so, some studies try to take advantage of varying natural experiments such as the extension of the electoral franchise (Batinti et al., 2019). In defining what democracy stands for, it is also possible to identify types of democracies. For example, one can identify the concept of 'anocracy', a regime characterised by 'intermediate' levels of democracies, which include 'soft dictatorships'. Furthermore, among democracies, one can distinguish different degrees of quality. Rosenberg and Shvetsova (2016) argue that the healthcare policy of autocracies is a core part of their wider economic policy, and targets, developing the labour force as a production factor. They show that autocracies manage to deal relatively well with those diseases most prevalent in the workforce. In contrast, democracies do not seem to show such a 'pro-labour' bias; their policy priorities depend on the preferences of the winning coalitions for the dimension of 'health' they find to be more salient (those visible to the PC).

Studies that identify an association between democracy and health typically employ measures of health outcomes such as mortality rates – especially infant and child rates per 1,000 live births used as proxies for human development, and others such as life expectancy rates, as well as measures of subjective well-being.[2] Evidence reveals significant heterogeneity across different measures, which indicates that democracy affects some dimensions of health more than others. Similarly, in measuring democracy, one can refer to different dimensions. A commonly used measure of democracy is employed by Boix, Miller and Rosato (Boix et al., 2013; BMR13),[3] who provide a dichotomous coding of democracies along the lines of measures originally proposed by Przeworski et al. (2000). The BMR13 index operationalises a measure of democracy according to the following criteria: the first is the adoption of a 'minimalistic' approach defining democracy, which codes as a democracy only if the necessary conditions for one exist. This follows the definition proposed in Dahl (1971). In contrast, this definition includes only two 'necessary' conditions: (i) there must be political contestation, for example decisions are taken through voting in free and fair elections; (ii) there must be political enfranchisement measured by a minimal level of suffrage. This is usually set to at least 50 per cent of the adult male population having the right to vote.[4] Finally, a common approach has been the construction of composite measures of democracy.[5]

---

[2] Part of the reason is that most of the gains in health during the first part of the twentieth century – gains in life expectancy – were mostly concentrated in reduction in mortality at young ages. Today other metrics should be used, as for example life expectancy at sixty-five or older ages, as recent gains in life expectancy might have been due mostly to reduction in mortality at old ages.

[3] The paper also discusses and compares the pros and cons of a wide series of alternative/complementary measures of democracy.

[4] One important alternative to the democracy index (BMR13) is the polity2 score from the Polity4 dataset. This is a multidimensional measure, which aggregates several dimensions and produces an index spanning from −10 (autocracy) to 10 (democracy). The resulting multicategory variable is thus not based on the minimal criteria proposed by Dahl (1971). For example, part of the index is built on adding a variable measuring social conflict, thus providing a very comprehensive definition of democracy, which must be used carefully. See, for example, Vreeland (2008) on the risk of an inappropriate use of the polity index when looking at the relationship between democracy as measured with polity data and conflict.

[5] This has been recently applied by Acemoglu, Naidu, Restrepo and Robinson (Acemoglu et al., 2019; ANRR), who use a wider number of sources to classify a given country as a democracy or not, and then code democracies when a certain agreement across sources is reached. Another approach uses machine-learning algorithms and compares several sources (Gründler and Krieger, 2018).

What Is the Evidence Linking Democracy and Health?

To better inform the discussion of the literature that can be seen over the next few pages, we provide here a set of figures displaying some 'stylised facts' about the temporal dynamics of the spread of democracy across the world. For this purpose, we use two dichotomous indicators, one from ANRR (2019), and the other is the polity2 score from the Polity4 dataset, which is normalised to 0. The y-axis of Figure 5.1 reports the percentage of countries classified as democracies; similar trends are detected both for the ANRR and Polity indexes, with some discrepancies especially between the 1970s and 1990s.

As the classification adopted in ANRR (2019) includes polity as well, we should expect any deviation to be explained by discrepancies in the way of classifying a democracy between polity2 and the other sources used in ANRR (2019). However, in both cases, we see a sharp increase in the percentage of democratic countries between the late 1980s and late 1990s, which is in significant part explained by the

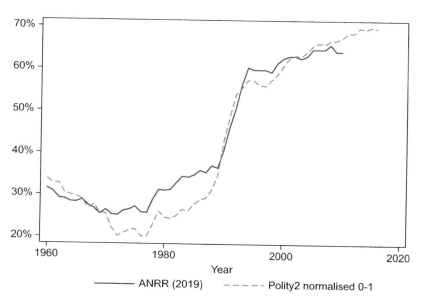

FIGURE 5.1 Spread of democracy (% of countries) across the world (1960–2015)
Note: ANRR is the dichotomous index created by using several sources. See ANRR (2019) for details on how it is calculated

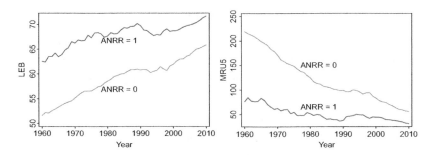

FIGURE 5.2 Dynamics of health differentials between democracies and non-democracies
Note: LEB = life expectancy at birth; MRU5 = mortality rate under five years old

collapse of the Soviet Union. After this, the trends are quite similar and show a slowdown in the democratisation process. Passing to the 'dependent' variables of interest, Figure 5.2 shows the distinct trends in life expectancy at birth and mortality for the population under five years old.

A breakdown of trends for the two subsets of democracies and non-democracies is shown. The figures show a democratic advantage in terms of health outcomes, though the difference wanes with time, especially in the case of the mortality index. In the case of life expectancy, we find evidence of common trends between democracies and non-democracies, though the life expectancy gap has remained quite substantial (about seven years' difference) and virtually constant in the last ten to fifteen years or so. As recently found in Bollyky et al. (2019), this can be partly explained by democracies being more effective in dealing with non-communicable disease, while consistent reductions in communicable disease have been observed both in democracies and autocracies. The latter likely also benefit from global health interventions mainly targeting communicable disease in low-income and autocratic regimes.[6]

---

[6] For completeness, we note this paper also uses an alternative definition of democracy, one coming from the Varieties of Democracies dataset. Please see Chapter 3 on the challenges for global health collective action.

In the remainder of the chapter, we propose a review of the literature aimed at testing the robustness of the stylised facts we have just shown with raw data. In particular, we discuss the possible mediating factors between democracy and health, and the findings, trying to infer if there is a causal nexus from democracy to health.

MECHANISMS AND MEDIATING FACTORS

The effect that democracy has on health is likely to be mediated by several factors. Below we identify and describe some of the main ones discussed in previous empirical research.

Stable versus Non-stable Democratic Transitions

Democratic transitions are heterogeneous because many countries have historically experienced setbacks from democracy back to autocracy throughout history. Hence, one ought to distinguish *stable* as opposed to *non-stable* democracies. A common claim is that it is only in stable democracies that health effects are identified, while countries subject to reversals or multiple changes in the democratic status may pay for this political instability with *worse* health outcomes than autocracies. Rather than a democratic transition, it is democratic stability and democratic duration that affect human development. Being young democracies with a higher risk of reversals, importance is placed on the capacity for a democracy to deliver a long-term and stable political and institutional environment which will produce more time-consistent policies. So, there will be some lag before observing significant results on human development and health. In other terms, it is not democratisation per se that is affecting human development as much as the years a country spent under a democratic regime. Young democracies tend to be overloaded by the management and extension of public programmes, if not supported by institutional quality and competent bureaucracies for implementation of programmes.

Furthermore, weak effective mechanisms of decision-making might make a health care crisis more problematic to be solved in young democracies. This argument is related to the modernisation hypothesis. It contends that only transitions occurring jointly with appropriate preconditions for democracy assure a long-lasting stable regime. Typically, democratic overload and policy non-reactivity might also be present in sclerotic democracies which are captured by powerful interest groups (Olson, 1965), and thus produce policies that fail in improving the human development of the population while redistributing to organised interests (see Chapter 9).

A subtler point refers to the long- and short-term value of democratisation. For example, political stability might work more in the long term through building quality in healthcare delivery, which is arguably a time-consuming process. Simultaneously, there might be short-term effects as well, through other types of mechanisms. Democratisation might be nested in the psychological effect of 'being freer' or expressing oneself through free and independent political participation, which gives rise to better health, including mental health (Benz and Frey, 2008). However, more democratic control of the government by giving voice to a broader number of views, might reduce corruption and waste (see Chapter 8) and enhance the checks and balances of political actions, might improve access to health inputs, including medicines and medical devices.

Inequality and Redistribution

Democracy transfers *de jure* political power to the 'median voter', who might vote based on its financial self-interest. When the median voter is relatively poorer than average (because income is right skewed and unequal) one would expect a higher demand for redistributive programmes, other things being equal. In such a scenario, public healthcare programmes are meant to improve the health of lower income people, and aim at furthering redistribution and access to healthcare. This is consistent with a Meltzer and

Richard (1981) type of median voter model. However, we note first that healthcare might have insurance purposes too, especially when referring to the fact that curative medicine is not achieved by public programmes through pure monetary redistribution, but instead it results from publicly provided health insurance itself or directly through the provision of health goods and services. In this case, there may be political equilibria where the median voter results from an alliance between rich and poor citizens against further expansion of such types of programmes (Epple and Romano, 1996a, 1996b). On this, see Chapter 6.

Second, it is important to stress that larger public health expenditures (in terms of GDP or total health expenditures, depending on the research question of interest), are not necessarily positively associated with better health outcomes if these are mis-directed and/or spent inefficiently (see evidence of this in Ross, 2006 and also the discussion in Part IV of this book). Hence, it is necessary to distinguish between indicators of healthcare systems outcomes and indicators of healthcare activity. While democratic transitions increase health expenditures, both the share of public expenditures (as a percentage of GDP) and the ratio between public and private expenditures have a moderate effect on health outcomes, even though they might impact quality of care.

Welfare Migration

As democracies become more attractive, migration tends to change the demographic composition of a country, leading perhaps to a change in the mortality/life expectancy of the host country. As migration happens for economic, political or health reasons, part of the migrant population might be expected to be in worse conditions than the population of the host country. However, very often the evidence indicates the opposite. The so-called 'healthy migrant effect' suggests that migrants tend to be healthier than the average host population, despite immigrants tending to come from countries with worse access to healthcare (Markides, 1983; Sorlie et al., 1993; Newbold, 2005). However, evidence comes from a small set of countries such as the United States and Canada, and might not be necessarily the case for all host countries.

Agency Alignment

Another explanation for a health value of democracies is that democracies select 'better' politicians, or they might be just more accountable and responsive to the demands of the median voter. Hence, then public spending might be better directed to the provision of public goods (for example, infrastructures of sanitation) which in turn might have significant health effects on the portion of the population that is more at risk.

The Political Role of Women and Female Enfranchisement

An important feature with respect to the political selection in democracies, is the progressive involvement of the female population in politics. Female enfranchisement ('votes for women') exerts two effects, namely a direct one of passive female participation, and a wider one of encouraging active participation in political life ('women can rule') both of which can have an impact on health through different mechanisms. The evidence from the literature suggests clear health gains from political involvement of the female population. Similarly, some studies find that female political empowerment has significant positive effects on several indicators of child health (Chattopadhyay and Duflo, 2004; Miller, 2008; Varkey et al., 2010; Swiss et al., 2012; Bhalotra and Clots-Figueras, 2014; Batinti et al., 2019).

Spread of Knowledge and Innovation

According to Angus S. Deaton (2004, p. 109): 'health improvement ultimately came from the globalization of knowledge, facilitated by local political, economic, and educational conditions'. That is, as democracy favours the circulation of scientific knowledge, it is likely to be conducive to improvements in medical effectiveness through medical innovation and its diffusion. As democracies allow a freer circulation of information, knowledge and scientific education, this was conductive to a more effective education on health behaviours. Also, as democracies are more likely to nurture a free press, their governments can be more responsive in intervening in times of health crisis (such as famine or earthquakes) because the circulation of information about crisis is more likely to circulate to the central government for intervention (Gao et al., 2017).

Civil Society, Psychosocial Factors and Overcoming of Collective Action

Civil Society and Social Capital

Democracy can stimulate the development of civil society and voluntary associations, as well as forms of social capital that can help improve the quality of life of citizens. A democratic government is more likely to delegate its functions to civil bodies of citizens that self-organise to promote social welfare. It also tends to be more tolerant of the specific demands of civil society and non governmental organisation that might promote specific health goals.

Subjective Well-Being

Another possible effect of democracy on health lies in improving subjective health status of the population (Frey and Stutzer, 2000; Inglehart et al., 2008; Altman et al., 2017; Loubser and Steenekamp, 2017). The latter, can influence physical health as a result.

WHAT DOES THE EVIDENCE TELL US?

The Positive Association between Democracy and Health

The evidence on the association between democracy and health is contentious. An early study using a cross-sectional sample of countries finds a positive association (Lena and London, 1993). Similar results are found in Frey and Al-Roumi (1999), and was also found

by Zweifel and Navia (2000). They found that political regimes classified as democracies do exhibit lower infant mortality rates and longer
life expectancy.

More recently, Franco et al. (2004) use the Freedom House
democracy index to examine the effect of democracy on life expectancy, maternal and infant mortality for a cross-sectional sample of
170 countries. They found a positive association between democracy
and the three health-status indicators mentioned. Similarly, Besley
and Kudamatsu (2006) document an effect by measuring outcomes in
terms of life expectancy at birth and infant mortality (other measures
are used in robustness checks, such as immunisation rates and clean
water supply).

More recently, Klomp and DeHaan (2009) offer both a review
of the literature and report results by using a cross-section of worldwide countries.[7] They apply factor analysis and individuate four
factors using multiple data sources. Indicators originating from
the principal component analysis are provided for (i) individual
health outcomes; (ii) healthcare sector quality; (iii) political regime
(democratic); and (iv) political stability. They then use structural
equation modelling, with the main findings showing that
democracy is positively associated with individual well-being. This
is a factor variable including mortality rates, a set of disease inci-
dences, vaccination rates and life expectancy. Second, they find that
income plays a mediating role. Moreover, regime instability is
negatively associated with individuals' health. Finally, Kudamatsu
(2012), which uses infant mortality as an indicator of health outcomes. Importantly, the paper finds that democratisation in sub-
Saharan Africa helped in reducing mortality rates (an average reduction of 1.8 percentage points). Similarly, a recent study using

---

[7] The paper also provides robustness tests using a panel of countries and Granger-type
causality test where political factors are measured with variables collected for a
period preceding the one used to collect variables for factors measuring individual
health and healthcare institutions.

Synthetic Control Analysis supports the view that democratisation has a positive effect by reducing infant mortality (Pieters et al., 2016) and the incidence of non-communicable disease (Bollyky et al., 2019).

Lack of Association

There is also research finding weak or no positive association between democracy and health. Houweling et al. (2005) use a sample cross-section of forty-three countries that focuses solely on developing countries. The health indicator in this paper is under-five (child) mortality rates. Their measure of democracy is based on the dataset provided initially in Easterly and Levine (1997). They find a positive, but not significant democratic effect. Consistently, Ross (2006) uses a panel of countries with averaged data and a yearly one with data filled by imputation. The main measures for health outcomes are child and infant mortality alongside two measures of democracy, and they find no significant effect of democracy on health. Ross (2006) reports two main explanations. The first is based on the inclusion, in the sample, of a series of relatively wealthy and healthy non-democracies (Organization of the Oil Exporting Countries (OPEC) countries) that were omitted in previous papers. The second reason is that the standard median voter prediction, based on the Meltzer and Richard (1981) model, and according to which democratisation should drive more redistribution of resources to the poorer, might just not hold if elites in democracies are organised so to distort the direction of redistribution towards the wealthier or to selected constituencies.

Mixed Findings

Finally, a number of studies find results that suggest mixed findings. Gerring et al. (2012) is a paradigmatic example. Child mortality rates are used as indexes of health and human development. The key contribution of this paper is that it distinguishes between *proximal and distal* causal effect of democracy on health outcomes. The authors found no evidence for the proximal effect, but a strong positive association for the distal effect. The latter is tested by using a *stock* definition of democracy calculated as taking a country's score from 1900 to the present year and applying a 1 per cent depreciation rate afterward.[8]

The progressive availability of new data might help in providing more convincing proof of the causality of the relationship. For example, Mackenback and McKee (2013)[9] exploits the two waves of democratisation and political reform in Europe. The first wave of democratisation involved Spain, Portugal and Greece in the 1970s, the second involved Central and Eastern Europe in the early 1990s. The paper finds mixed results and, like Gerring et al. (2012), also distinguishes between two distinct sub-periods, 1960–90 and 1987–2008, which produced the following two sets of results: (i) the period 1960–90 using current democracy finds a strong positive association with life expectancy and negative association with overall mortality; the last one mediated by specific causes of mortality – heart disease is one of those. (ii) As already said, for the period 1987–2008, current democracy is instead associated with *lower* life expectancy, and cumulative democracy with longer life expectancy. Important mediating factors when a cumulative democracy is used are cancer and circulatory disease. Results are overall mixed and, generally, the existence of a causal relationship (Acemoglu et al., 2015) is hard to prove. Such challenges are theoretically exposed in the *modernisation hypothesis* (Lipset, 1959), which sees democratisation as the joint contribution of economic, social and political factors, which in turn can

---

[8] The paper strongly relies on data imputation for several variables, and basically the *stock* definition of democracy is a way to proxy countries' fixed effects.

[9] Several measures of democratisation waves have been utilised in the literature about democracy. We report only Mackenback and McKee (2013) because, to our knowledge, it is the first study to utilise this identification strategy using health measures as dependent variables.

affect health outcomes in a society.[10] The omission of any of these factors could create an estimation bias with the risk of reaching misleading conclusions. If so, usual metrics of social and economic development, such as per capita GDP and education, would affect democratisation as well as health status (Grossman, 1972a, 1972b).

EFFECTS ON HEALTH INEQUALITY

Democracy can potentially reduce health inequalities by prioritising programmes that improve the health of the neediest. The more democratic a society is, with re-election incentives guiding political competition, the more responsive politicians will be to popular demands calling for further investments in public health, and more generally social programmes that address health needs of more deprived populations (Holmberg and Rothstein, 2011). For example, by promoting equal rights and protection for all groups under the law, regardless of socio-economic status, gender, age or ethnicity, one would expect to see an effect on the health distribution of the population (Mann et al., 1994). Similarly, a closer representation of the poorest members of society (Mulligan et al., 2004) is likely to give rise to the introduction of new health programmes enhancing the safety net of the poorest in society (Acemoglu and Robinson, 2000; Krueger et al., 2015), mainly because it strengthens the political power of poorer segments of society, which would increase support for more redistributive programmes (Acemoglu et al., 2018). Acemoglu and Robinson (2005) refer to the process of political selection, with democracies having more transparent mechanisms to

---

[10] This is not the only perspective. A contrasting one is the view of *critical junctures* (institutions first) as proposed in Acemoglu et al. (2009). Here democratisation is seen as the product of historical critical junctures produced by exogenous events *plus* the establishment of specific institutions (productive instead of extractive) which have been conducive to democratic transition, and which, ultimately, caused socio-economic development.

select competent and honest executives. Finally, democracies tend to offer more universal access to healthcare (Oswald, 2013). Following this rationale, one would expect health inequality to be smaller in democracies. The prioritisation of both public health and redistribution would be expected to influence the association between income and health (and hence socio-economic inequalities), alongside pure health insurance.

Nonetheless, democracy can lead to a 'health-inequality trap' when it fails to deliver on the needs of minorities, and becomes captured by dominant elites (Powell-Jackson et al., 2011). If social cohesion in a society is low and, consequently, social division is high, the majority might not be interested in policy responses to deal with the health risks of minorities, leading to growing or at least persistent inequalities in health (Powell-Jackson et al., 2011, p. 34). If the elites, for example, manage to capture the political will of the middle class by whatever means, the government might be less redistributive (Acemoglu and Robinson, 2005). Second, some argue that democratic societies might not necessarily improve the health of the neediest (Krueger et al., 2015), but might focus instead on improving the health of the pivotal voters.

SUMMARY

The relationship between health and democracy is contentious. In this chapter we argue that the effect of democracy on health might be heterogeneous depending on a democracy's maturity, to the point that, as we have shown, some scholars hypothesise that what really matters is the distal versus proximal causal effect of democracy on health and human development. Another explanation is that democracies have often been introduced after long periods of social conflict and violence. Thus, health outcomes measured right before the introduction of democracy might well show a pre-transition dip. Furthermore, democracy changes the sequence of policymaking in healthcare, where initial interventions of sanitation, vaccination and other preventive healthcare measures might be the ones reaping most of the welfare effects, while the reactive nature of curative systems, illustrated the treatments to fight chronic diseases, might be the ones that contribute less to well-being and quality of life.

6 Theory of Political Markets in Healthcare

As we document in Chapter 1, as nations develop economically, healthcare becomes a major focus of government responsibility.[1] More specifically, in 2018, 60 per cent of Americans agreed on increasing federal healthcare government responsibility.[2] Across OECD countries, health expenditure is the most dynamic component of public expenditure. This expansion in government spending coincides with the democratisation of health systems, or the increasing collective decision-making in which patient citizens (PCs) indirectly (by electing the right representatives) make choices among competing projects. Such choice of PCs on the demand side is complemented with competition between Special Interest Groups (SIGs) in delimiting policies. In contrast, the supply side refers to the administrative procedures, ideological affiliation and other feature that define the selection of candidates and their policies.

In such a setting, a pivotal question to examine is how the PC policy preferences affect public healthcare spending. We argue that this takes place in what we call a 'political market', namely the political contests where several candidates compete for the support of constituents who, similarly as consumer in markets, exercise their 'political sovereignty'. More specifically, this chapter discusses how political markets work in healthcare as well as how preferences for healthcare policies are aggregated and influence policymaking through the election of representatives in assemblies and executive positions. We discuss how the institutional design of how voting takes place determines healthcare policies.

---

[1] www.commonwealthfund.org/sites/default/files/documents/___media_files_publications_fund_report_2017_may_mossialos_intl_profiles_v5.pdf.

[2] https://news.gallup.com/poll/4708/healthcare-system.aspx.

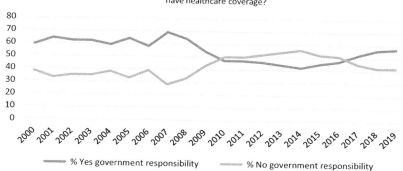

FIGURE 6.1 Responsibility for health insurance – government
responsibility role
Source: Gallup, several years

Figure 6.1 reports the self-reported perception of US citizens
with regards to the federal role in healthcare. Overall, there is a
majority supporting such a federal role except for the period 2010–14
where the Affordable Care Act (ACA) was discussed and appealed.

In this chapter, we outline several different explanations for
the selection of varied health policies *within* a democracy. Political
markets influence healthcare decisions and voters are interested in
building Wicksellian connections to understand how much they contribute to the public healthcare system, and what they can obtain
from it. Similarly, voters might have redistributive concerns, and
hence their political choices could be reflective of inequality aversion
in the domains of health and income.

Political economists typically use the median voter model as a
parsimonious departure point for theoretical analysis, which allows
understanding the dynamics of a democracy with PCs' policy preferences being single peaked or single-crossing policy preferences.[3] In such

---

[3] *Single-peaked preferences* are verified when each voter has an optimal policy, and
policies furtherly distant from the ideal one are progressively less and less preferred.
Single-crossing policy preferences are technically more challenging to define. We direct
the reader to Persson and Tabellini (2000) and Borck (2007) for an in-depth discussion.

a setting one would obtain the so-called standard median voter equilibrium model (MVM). If policy preferences can be mapped[4] into the income distribution, then the median voter will be the voter with median income. Thus, an increase in income inequality, widening the distance between the median and average income, should make the median voter demand more redistribution and hence public health spending will increase. However, comparing public health provision to mere redistribution is a strong assumption, as healthcare is often a publicly provided *private* good. In such circumstances, an alternative voter equilibrium is the so-called ends against the middle (EAM) where a coalition of rich and poor voters supports less health spending at the expense of the middle class. On the other hand, some authors have argued for the presence of a 'middle-class capture' for certain health policies (Costa-Font and Zigante, 2016), suggesting that the preferences of the middle class explain the significant reforms of healthcare systems, such as reforms expanding provider choice in the UK.

Finally, we discuss some of the limitations of the MVM, and refer to alternative explanations for drivers of health policymaking, such as the potential for collusion between different stakeholders. We also discuss other influences as to how political competition works, such as the effects of ideology, which keep the loyalty of individuals to a party (we return to this point in Chapter 7), as well as other important aspects, such as the gender of the incumbent which might play a role if psychosocial traits like empathy or simply a different set of priorities and life visions are incorporated in the political decision-making process (Bhalotra and Clots-Figueras, 2014), and beauty (Berggren et al., 2010).

We limit ourselves here to convey the intuition behind this regularity. Suppose we have three voters with low, medium and high income, respectively Vl, Vm and Vh. Suppose they have to vote between two tax rates, low and high Tl and Th. If Vm prefers Tl to Th, then Vh has to prefer Tl to Th. If Vm prefers Th to Tl, then Vl has to prefer Th to Tl. If this holds for all voters, then the median voter results apply as well. Note, single-crossing preferences do not necessarily have to be single-peaked.

[4] This would be the case, for example, with single-crossing preferences.

This chapter provides a self-contained introductory treatment on issues around the electoral politics of healthcare. We do not elaborate in detail about modelling assumptions and instead provide the intuition behind the theoretical reasoning in political economy as far as median voter models are concerned. Consistent with the general setting of this book, this chapter intend to supply a guide for further reading to those interested in a more in-depth and, perhaps, research-oriented understanding in the field of the political economy of health and healthcare.

THE POLITICAL DEMAND FOR HEALTHCARE

Central to this section is the median voter model (MVM), a model of spatial competition originally proposed in industrial organisation (Hotelling, 1929) and widely used as mainframe of electoral politics, at least since Smithies (1941), Bowen (1943), Black (1948) and Downs (1957a, 1957b). Typically, agents in political markets differ in one-dimensional policy, and politicians attempt to attract support of the majority of the voters which is obtained by supplying the policy preferred by the median voter.

As mentioned, the model introduces spatial competition in politics, divides between a supply and demand side of policies and results in an equilibrium solution of the competitive quest for political success. In its core formulation and most basic version, it is, however, most prominently a demand-side model, where the supply side – politicians – reacts automatically to voters' preferences to settle on the 'Condorcet Winner' (CW) policy, in other words the policy mostly preferred by the median voter. Thus, PCs can be thought of as indirectly *electing* policies.[5] Nonetheless, the MVM has restrictive assumptions. There are, as a result, extensions to the model which have attempted to make it more realistic. A complete review of all the models which have been proposed as alternatives or extensions to the

[5] For a recent survey on elect-versus-select models and an account of the critics of the MVM, see Padovano (2013).

MVM is beyond the scope of this chapter. Instead, we present an assessment of what types of models have been used to explain the electoral politics of healthcare. Although clearly the MVM cannot be considered the final approach to every possible policy question, it serves as a good departure point (Holcombe, 1989; Persson and Tabellini, 2000; Congleton, 2003; Mueller, 2003; Borck, 2007; Kifmann, 2009).

Let us begin with examining some data from OECD countries in Table 6.1. Panels A and B provide a picture suggesting three stylised facts. First, healthcare spending is growing in importance at the expense of other sources of social spending. Second, healthcare is overall the second-largest item after social protection (mostly pensions). However, third, it is the type of healthcare that exhibits the highest growth rates for the period across all sectors (Panel B).

Panels (A) and (B) in Table 6.1 show first that public health expenditure as a share of total public spending is second only with respect to social protection. However, health registered by and large the highest average percentage increase, +25.5 per cent from 1995 to 2010. Should this growth trend continue it will soon reach similar shares to that of pensions, which still account for between 70 and 80 per cent of total social protection in several OECD countries. Similar trends are to be expected for non-OECD, but fast-growing countries such as China. These trends pose important questions: what is responsible for such trends? If the government is taking an increasingly active role in healthcare decision-making, what are the institutional drivers of such a change? How political markets influence healthcare decisions?

THE MEDIAN VOTER EXPLANATION

In the median voter model (MVM) proposed in Romer (1975), Roberts (1977) and Meltzer and Richard (1981),[6] for brevity RRMR, the MVM is

---

[6] For this section, see also the review offered in Borck (2007), from which we heavily borrow, and also take the RRMR acronym.

Table 6.1 Shares of government spending by function of government (COFOG classification)

Country	020 Defence (%)	030 Public order and safety (%)	070 Health (%)	090 Education (%)	100 Social protection (overall) (%)
(A) Shares in 1995					
France	4.59	2.73	*13.01*	10.56	39.16
Germany	2.65	2.97	*11.17*	8.04	37.05
Italy	2.44	3.72	*10.21*	8.59	33.95
Norway	4.90	1.99	*14.01*	12.23	35.28
Spain	3.07	4.46	*11.84*	9.71	32.42
Sweden	3.71	2.17	*9.58*	10.98	40.23
United Kingdom	7.23	4.77	*13.05*	11.40	38.26
United States	10.06	5.21	*17.50*	15.89	19.44
(B) Shares in 2010					
France	3.30	2.98	*14.08*	9.98	41.87
Germany	2.30	3.35	*14.75*	9.21	42.12
Italy	2.65	4.05	*14.88*	8.76	39.80
Norway	3.26	2.13	*16.51*	11.70	38.69
Spain	2.28	4.74	*14.41*	9.83	36.34
Sweden	2.96	2.66	*13.22*	12.69	41.14
United Kingdom	5.39	5.26	*16.03*	13.58	35.64
United States	10.98	5.35	*20.54*	15.95	21.05

(Continued)

Table 6.1 (cont.)

Country	020 Defence (%)	030 Public order and safety (%)	070 Health (%)	090 Education (%)	100 Social protection (overall) (%)
(C) % Change in budget share					
France	−28.05	9.08	8.19	−5.49	6.94
Germany	−13.39	12.99	32.00	14.60	13.70
Italy	8.37	8.81	45.75	1.95	17.25
Norway	−33.47	6.78	17.85	−4.34	9.66
Spain	−25.52	6.41	21.78	1.28	12.07
Sweden	−20.08	22.73	38.05	15.63	2.27
United Kingdom	−25.50	10.30	22.78	19.16	−6.86
United States	9.14	2.81	17.38	0.39	8.27
Unweighted average % growth in budget shares	−16.06	9.99	25.47	5.40	7.91

Notes: Data sources: OECD. General government expenditures and selected COFOG sectors are: 010: General public services; 020: Defence; 030: Public order and safety; 040: Economic affairs; 050: Environmental protection; 060: Housing and community amenities; 070: Health; 080: Recreation, culture and religion; 090: Education; 100: Overall social protection. Accessed September 2017. Our calculations of growth rate (1995–2010) of shares by function of general government expenditures (C).

used to explain the size of government as the consequence of a political equilibrium, where the PC characterised by the median income is also the one supporting the CW level of redistribution. The size of government is measured by the amount of redistributive taxes.

The RRMR is an elegant and parsimonious attempt at providing a connection between the inequality of income distribution and the preferred level of redistribution expressed by voters' policy preferences. This model is quite intuitive and empirically testable. A common characteristic of the income distribution is its right-skewedness and, as a consequence, the median income stands below the mean income. If so, rising inequality, defined by a growing distance between the mean and median income, increases the demand for redistribution (and, hence, public healthcare spending), as the median voter is now relatively poorer than the average voter. The second result is, in the presence of an utilitarian welfare-maximiser government, that the tax applied would be the one preferred by the average voter, but the policy process would push the size of redistribution – and hence public healthcare programmes – beyond that level, towards a larger and suboptimal one, which is the one preferred by the voter with median income.

The empirical test of the theory has often been conducted by using the Gini index as a proxy for inequality, under the assumption that it would be positively correlated with the size of median–mean distance in incomes. This is clearly also a major assumption, as increases in the Gini index do not necessarily imply a growing distance between the mean and median income. Recently, more rigorous tests have been applied by using data from the Luxembourg Income Study (LIS). An early empirical exploration occurs in Milanovic (2000), which supports the RRMR hypothesis, while more recently, with updated data, Scervini (2012) fails to support the RRMR.

With progressively larger shares of public budgets directed to healthcare, health care scholars have examined whether this model is an appropriate formal tool to understand the dynamics observed in public health budgets. Overall, despite the lack of consistent empirical support, there is also reason to believe that a deterministic cash-transfers model cannot be considered adequate when looking at the political economy of healthcare. The original RRMR model has been extended to incorporate other features such as the existence of (i) uncertainty and insurance motives and, most of all, (ii) public provision of private goods, two key elements when considering an application in the case of healthcare.

Adding Uncertainty

One of the limitations of the RRMR approach to health politics is that the PC finds it less clear-cut to predict policy outcomes in health care, compared to cash benefits. Health policies are usually designed to combine both redistribution (e.g. improving access to the less well-off) and insurance (e.g. reducing the cost of expanding coverage for all individuals), and it is unclear whether all new public programmes improve redistribution (see Moene and Wallerstein, 2003). Moene and Wallerstein find three main implications.

The first two are, respectively, when insurance is offered only to the employed (pure redistribution) or only to the unemployed, in other words when the adverse condition of a job loss occurs (pure insurance). In the first case, the model replicates the predictions of the RRMR model. The reason is quite intuitive: in this way, the problem is reduced to an RRMR model, but among the portion of the population of wage earners.[7] When insurance is provided only to those who are jobless, however, an increase in inequality in the wage distribution corresponds to a smaller demand for insurance redistribution. In this case, a negative income effect prevails over the positive tax-price effect for the demand of insurance. The third case, referred to as being a close match to the health insurance case, is where government provides healthcare insurance, and where both wage earners and

---

[7] One assumption in the model is that those who are jobless are indifferent and vote randomly for any of the two candidates. However, had they preferences for global efficiency, they could vote for a zero tax rate to minimise deadweight losses from taxation. In that case the median voter in the population would be poorer than the median voter among wage earners, and potentially one favouring a zero tax rate.

unemployed people enjoy the same amount of redistribution. This is the case of a universal health coverage plan, where both employed and unemployed people are entitled to government-provided health insurance. In this case, results depend on individuals risk aversion. For values of relative risk aversion slightly above unity, the overall effect will be an increase in the preferred tax rate (and thus redistribution), while, as (relative) risk aversion approaches infinity, the effect turns negative, because again income effects offset the effects of the tax price.

This approach provides two insights as to how conditional redistributive incentives shape social insurance programmes. First, the model assumes health insurance to be unconditional on job status, which would be the case under a national healthcare system. It is, however, not unconditional regarding health status, and health risks are not explicitly modelled. While health insurance can arguably be unconditional on job risks, it is not so for health risks. Second, health systems do not provide only insurance, but in many cases, governments prefer in-kind publicly provided private health goods and services for citizens.

EXTENSIONS INVOLVING HEALTHCARE SUPPLY

The economics literature has devoted specific attention to goods like healthcare that can be provided by the market but are publicly funded. Epple and Romano (1996a, 1996b) and Gouveia (1997) explore the political equilibria when healthcare, a private good, is provided through public funding. We note first that an important part of healthcare is curative medicine supplied *in kind* by public services. This suggests that, in many instances, governments publicly provide private goods. Table 6.2 shows that curative medicine, expressed as a percentage of total current public expenditures on health, is much larger than preventive care.

With reference to the public provision of private goods, Stiglitz (1974) showed that, when private alternatives are not available, there is no voting equilibrium. This occurs when here is no option of private supplementation, be it out-of-pocket or through private insurance. We

Table 6.2 *Composition of public healthcare spending*

Country	Curative rehab.	LT	Prev.	Country	Curative rehab.	LT	Prev.
Australia	49.17	1.75	1.79	Japan	51.01	14.67	1.79
Austria	47.87	11.84	1.50	Korea	28.29	9.70	2.78
Belgium	37.02	20.64	1.61	Luxembourg	45.72	17.82	2.04
Canada	41.13	11.37	6.01	Netherlands	41.39	23.79	2.92
Denmark	48.32	22.16	2.31	Norway	43.09	25.80	2.38
Finland	47.00	15.03	2.10	Poland	48.59	5.83	1.68
France	46.14	10.53	1.36	Portugal	47.70	1.66	0.86
Germany	46.43	10.68	2.75	Spain	44.02	7.63	2.07
Iceland	47.47	19.86	2.26	Sweden	47.21	21.50	2.55
Ireland	36.85	17.58	1.66	Switzerland	32.67	13.29	1.28
Israel	48.92	5.65	0.22	United Kingdom	50.30	12.27	3.99
Italy	45.69	7.82	3.36	United States	34.17	3.36	2.86

Notes: Selected OECD countries: measures are percentage shares of current expenditure on health, averages 2010–16; all providers financing through government/compulsory schemes. Functions: (i) Curative and rehabilitative care; (ii) Long-term care (health); (iii) Preventive care. Functions not included: Ancillary services (non-specified by function); Governance and health system and financing administration; Medical goods (non-specified by function). LT = Long-Term Care.

note, however, that health systems only rarely do not allow private supplementation, and they tend to be heterogeneous in terms of expenditure types. They are often the result of the interplay of several sources of financing and spending, those being private or public (Besley and Gouveia, 1994; Congleton et al., 2017). Table 6.3 shows, in fact, that private alternatives, both pursued through out-of-pocket spending or recurring to private insurance, are also non-trivial parts of health spending in OECD countries with National Health Services.

THE 'ENDS AGAINST THE MIDDLE' EXPLANATION

The political influence in the supply of healthcare goods and services in the presence of private alternatives has more nuanced equilibrium results (Epple and Romano, 1996a, 1996b; Gouveia, 1997). In the presence private health insurance or out-of-pocket purchase of healthcare goods and services in the private market, one important theoretical contribution is the possibility of an 'ends against the middle' (EAM) political equilibrium.[8] In fact three equilibria are possible. First, an RRMR-type equilibrium, one where the voter with median characteristic (income) is the pivotal one, is still possible. Second, an EAM equilibrium is possible as well. A Crucial assumption for this result is that the private good must be a normal good (i.e. a good whose demand increases with income) and that there is an option for private provision. There is significant evidence that the consumption of health goods and services responds positively to income increases. In particular, this equilibrium happens when the income effect of public provision is stronger than the costs of extra taxes paid by for part of the population. In other words, given a certain income level, the tax price will be so large that the rich will prefer zero public provision, and will opt out of the public and turn into private provision. At the same time the poor might have similar policy

---

[8] This alternative can come both with the possibility of supplementing out-of-pocket or through recurring to private insurance. Perfect substitution between private and public is also assumed, and no uncertainty and asymmetric information.

Table 6.3 *Composition of household health spending*

Country	Private insurance	Household out-of-pocket payments	Country	Private insurance	Household out-of-pocket payments
Australia	12.31	19.63	Japan	3.12	13.22
Austria	6.31	17.94	Korea	5.95	37.32
Belgium	4.52	18.07	Luxembourg	6.53	10.50
Canada	14.95	14.71	Netherlands	7.43	11.05
Denmark	1.92	13.96	New Zealand	7.14	12.63
Finland	5.88	19.31	Norway	0.35	14.72
France	14.33	7.19	Portugal	6.07	26.89
Germany	2.91	13.36	Spain	4.95	22.90
Iceland	1.46	17.74	Sweden	1.09	15.60
Ireland	13.35	13.79	Switzerland	8.37	27.84
Israel	12.60	23.43	United Kingdom	6.49	12.43
Italy	1.81	21.83	United States	39.42	11.80

Notes: Selected OECD countries. Measure: Share of current expenditure on health, unweighted average 2010–16. Provider counting all providers. Financing scheme. Voluntary healthcare payment schemes and Household out-of-pocket payments. Function: Current expenditure on health (all functions).

preferences to the rich, but for different reasons (including that they can still benefit from a means tested system). For the poor, the negative income effect is stronger than the positive price (tax) effect for public provision, with the result being again a very low demand for public provision. Finally, there will be an intermediate alternative, where the demand for the public provision of the private good increases with the income of middle-class voters. This effect might be exacerbated by the presence of high inequality, in which case a coalition of poor and rich supporting a very low level of public provision is possible, which gives rise to the so-called ends against the middle. Thus, the relationship between inequality and the level of public provision would be exactly the opposite of the one expected in the RRMR model.

While there is ample empirical literature testing the RRMR hypothesis, there seem to be fewer empirical exercises trying to test EAM equilibrium, at least in healthcare. Kotakorpi and Laamanen (2010) match public healthcare spending of Finnish municipalities with individual satisfaction, finding that middle-income people are more satisfied with increasing spending, but this is not so for either low- or high-income individuals. This evidence seems to be at least consistent with an EAM political equilibrium.

RECENT CONTRIBUTIONS AND EXTENSIONS

Successive contributions have focused more on information problems of health insurance systems, such as moral hazard and adverse selection. Also, in these cases the possible equilibria options remain the same, confirming the robustness of the results in Epple and Romano (1996a, 1996b). Anderberg (1999) proposes a similar setting, where public health insurance can be supplemented by private health insurance and there is *adverse selection* in the private market.[9] Again, while both RRMR and EAM equilibria are possible, the numerical

---

[9] To be precise the example developed takes pensions as a reference, but the model can be adapted to one with provision of health insurance. Another interesting paper developing adverse selection in the framework of Gouveia (1997) is Delipalla and O'Donnell (1999).

example provided by the author shows that RRMR equilibria are more likely to occur when individuals are heterogeneous on risk types, and EAM is more likely to occur when heterogeneity is instead based on income differences. The two heterogeneities are then analysed separately. Intuition helps in understanding why this can be the case. With adverse selection, insurance premia reflect more high-risk types, so that low-risk individuals will pay disproportionately with respect to their type in a pooled insurance contract. When individuals are heterogenous by income, the high prices faced in the private market can overcome the high premia paid in the form of taxes to the government. So, and with respect to a private alternative offering fair premia, high-income voters will tend to prefer the public solution to the private. This makes an RRMR equilibrium more likely to exist, because an EAM equilibrium can exist only if there is a consistent group of high-income voters preferring zero public provision and opting out.

Casamatta et al. (2000) studies a two-stage constitutional choice, where at the first stage it is decided whether there is a social insurance entailment or if the health system is funded by general taxation, and at the second stage the politically viable tax rate to finance the system chosen in the first stage is voted for. The model produces four insights. One is the occurrence of a suboptimal redistributive system, which is arranged to ensure the political support in the second stage of the collective choice process. Second, private insurance crowds out public insurance. On the other hand, supplementary private insurance may increase the welfare of the poor, even if it is effectively bought only by the rich. Finally, there may be political equilibria where the majority of the voters prefer prohibiting access to supplementary private insurance as the efficiency of private insurance markets increases.

Alternatively, Kifmann (2005) adopts a two-stage modelling approach, where at the constitutional stage voters choose unanimously whether to adopt a public health insurance system or not. As a result, the rich segment of the population will also agree on such a system to be financed through income-related taxes. This is because private insurance markets are incomplete and do not offer insurance against a risk premium while a public system does. De Donder and

Hindricks (2007) propose an alternative to the median voter model, where there are two parties (Left and Right) maximising the utility of their members/voters. Within this framework, the political equilibrium depends on the whole range of the two distributions of risk types and income. One result is that more income inequality does not necessarily imply a higher demand for social insurance, and that in a context of a more polarised income distribution, both parties can in fact propose *less* social insurance.

In another contribution, Moreno-Ternero and Roemer (2010) propose alternative equilibrium concepts, including a multidimensional space, where candidates are policy-oriented and not merely office-seeking. In modeling healthcare spending, voters can be thought of voting not only depending on their location in the income distribution, but also on the base of their ideologies.[10] In Li et al. (2016) the private-public mix of health expenditures chosen in a political equilibrium is made to depend on the substitutability between private and public healthcare and the respective effects of public and private spending on voters' survival probabilities. Finally, Kifmann and Roeder (2018) discuss the political support of social health insurance schemes and their relative substitutability or complementarity resulting from a political equilibrium.

New theoretical approaches have been crafted to consider essential elements in healthcare, such as technological progress,[11] as technology is found to be a main driver of healthcare benefits and cost (Weisbrod, 1991; Newhouse, 1992; Okunade and Murthy, 2002; Murphy and Topel, 2003a, 2006; Chandra and Skinner, 2012; and Chapter 10 of this book). The technological dimension has been incorporated in at least two papers. Bethencourt and Galasso (2008) explore the political interdependency of social security and public health

---

[10] This aspect has been brought to attention, though from different perspectives, in previous research (Potrafke, 2010; Congleton et al., 2011).

[11] As multidimensional policy is inherently unstable (Plott, 1967), often models use the idea of a structured-induced equilibrium, as proposed in Shepsle (1979). Structured-induced equilibria solutions are possible because there is a breakdown of the policy problem in sequential choices, one dimension at a time.

spending. As health spending fosters longevity, it also increases social security spending. Therefore, an exogenous change in health technology – which increases public health spending productivity – has the effect of strengthening the mutual interdependence of the two public programmes. Finally, Batinti and Congleton (2018) propose a median voter model exploring the electoral interdependency of the political support of health R&D, technology and public healthcare programmes.

GEROTOCRACY AND MIDDLE-CLASS CAPTURE

It is possible to argue that other models could also explain healthcare activity. One is the increasing role of an ageing population, and specifically the coalition of middle-aged and older-age individuals in setting the health policy agenda (gerontocracy). This argument follows on from Tabellini (2000). An alternative argument lies in the existence of a middle-class capture of the health system. This explanation assumes that the supply of health policies would not cater to the entire electorate but to the demands of the middle class. This point has been extended and documented in Costa-Font and Zigante (2016) to expand provider choice in healthcare and was previously made by Goodin and Le Grand (1987). Other important approaches that shift the political market for healthcare include the role of media in reporting about dimensions of healthcare that individuals use to judge their health systems, such as waiting times and lists, hospital closures and other proxies of quality, as well as measures of coverage, such as the introduction or exclusion of cost-sharing and negative lists of health programmes limiting and delisting services covered by the health system.

SUMMARY

This chapter has discussed the literature on the electoral politics of healthcare. As health spending, and especially its public component, has increased dramatically across countries, it has become an object of interest for general interest politics types of models such as the median voter models. We have listed some of the theoretical models including the median voter model (MVM) in the Romer Roberts

Meltzer Richard (RRMR) version, the 'ends against the middle' (EAM) voter equilibrium and, finally, the middle-class capture (MCC) and gerontocracy approaches. We have argued also that limits and barriers to political participation can influence electoral outcomes. If richer patient citizens are most likely to vote, the median voter is likely to support less redistribution and will limit the growth of the public health system (for a recent survey on the topic see Borck, 2018).

While progress has been made, we need to take into account that health systems tend to be complex institutional conglomerates whose role may be obscured by testing general models of government spending. This is surely a challenge that must be undertaken by future research. For example, public supply might be chosen in terms of in-kind instead of insurance provision. Private insurance might be allowed to supplement or complement the public one, which is typically the results of differences in perceived quality (Besley et al., 1999; Costa-Font and Garcia, 2003). Those who do not wish to use the public system might be allowed to do so or not, although this might have a deteriorating effect on the quality of the public system. If private insurance is allowed, the PC might still be required to pay their share of taxes and dues to the government (supplementary insurance), or might be allowed to opt out with tax discounts as the PC is not using the public health system (under substitutive insurance). However, opt-outs, even when only partial, have two effects. They decongest the system in the short run, but might reduce the support for public insurance in the longer run (Costa-Font and Jofre-Bonet, 2008). Whether one effect or the other prevails is an empirical question that is influenced by the role of different ideologies, the transparency in the political process, as well as the extent of rent-seeking and corruption, as we discuss in Part IV of the book.

7   Ideology and Healthcare

A large body of the literature in social sciences has documented the influence of ideas on public policymaking. Policy innovation, policy transfer and imitation have been carefully examined for more than two decades (Rose, 2004). However, the evidence on how ideas influence health policymaking and the role of the different stakeholders is rarely included in the standard theoretical approaches of the political economy of health systems. This chapter will attempt to bring together some of these contributions, and identify the specific links with the political economy literature.

With respect to healthcare, policymaking often takes different channels than in other sectors, mostly due to its specialised nature. This provides additional power to medical associations and professionals groups alongside specific interest groups (insurance companies as well as the industries producing medicines and medical devices). This influence extends to the agendas of agents competing in the electoral process, alongside lobbyists interested in specific healthcare policy outcomes.

Political agendas reveal priorities between competing health programmes that health systems are potentially considering. They are often reflected in the extent of reimbursement (e.g. the introduction of co-payments) of certain programmes and more generally in the distribution of expenditures (e.g. pharmaceutical treatments versus preventive programmes) and status of different specialisations within healthcare organisations (e.g. surgeons versus paediatricians).

Political agendas defining the process of electoral competition can take the form of traditional party groupings (e.g. liberal, social-democratic, socialist, green, conservative, nationalist). However, political agendas do not always coincide with effective influence in reducing inequality, let alone in improving health of the population, or the size of the public budgets.

This chapter examines the role of the influence of political ideologies, both of the patient citizen (PC) and that of decision makers (supply side), in the form of competition in the electoral market alongside the influence of different interest groups in healthcare reform. We specifically examine the unique aspects of healthcare decision-making and how political influences can happen. We will then document an association between health and the political cycle, as well as provide a summary of the existing evidence on the effect of political influences on health.

'LEFT' AND 'RIGHT' HEALTH POLICY

Policymaking in health, as in other areas, takes off when stakeholders propose reform ideas. Such ideas commonly boil down to institutional responses to an unsolved problem (e.g. limited competition, too many uninsured people, limited prevention), as well as the need to address the adverse consequences of a new technology, among others. Ideological conceptions in health policymaking determine what the ideal health system should look like, which affects both the demand and supply of health policies. On the supply side of the political market, political ideologies are presented as slogans of what should be the goal of a policy (e.g. access for all, no barrier to care, etc.). They are narratives to attract attention, which are upheld by policymaking elites in setting policy goals, and narratives that justify the policies. Slogans are reciprocated by political ideologies which underpin political manifestos and popular political culture based on the demand side.

Ideologies can range from conservative to liberal or socialist. Competing political views differ across many dimensions: the weight they place on competition and the market mechanism in the allocation of goods and services within the healthcare markets, the size of public intervention, the role the government should play in improving equality of opportunity and in reducing inequality of outcomes. Ideological differences are then reflected in policy choices such as the priority that competition has in driving healthcare delivery, or the level of autonomy of healthcare providers, as well as the role of fairness in the financing of healthcare and the precedence of health improvement of underprivileged individuals in society. More generally, differences across health systems reflect the inequality aversion of the population in the system. Countries also vary in whether the right to healthcare is constitutionally established. Clearly, liberals and conservatives will put more emphasis on the role of markets in the allocation of goods and services, including the provision of healthcare and its insurance. At the opposite end of the political spectrum, socialist parties will put more emphasis on the role of the State in solving market failures, and they will be somewhat averse to too much competition, which can reduce quality in the presence of asymmetric information, and will be worried by private insurance companies, which can skim the market and select customers. Left and right, socialist and liberal, are of course different concepts in different countries. The absence of a strong communist party in the USA clearly characterises Republican and Democrats in a different way with respect to left and right parties in Europe, with clear consequences as to how the previous categories are represented. Ideologies are very much context dependent, and serve the purpose of differentiating both the demand and supply participants in political markets.

These differences aside, under a standard partisan political process, left of centre parties are more likely to support policies that increase the size of the (public) healthcare sector, and hence prioritise health expenditure above other policy areas. Such expansionary policies tend to have the support of the middle classes which, in turn, demand quality improvement such as provider choice in the context of national health systems (Costa-Font and Zigante, 2016). De Donder and Hindriks (2007) examine the political economy of social insurance policy and demonstrate that in a two-party model, the left-wing party proposes more social insurance than the right-wing party. The right-wing party attracts the richer voters, and voters with smaller health risks, and the left-wing party attracts the poorer voters, and voters with higher health risks. As a result, the leftist party appeals more to the labour base and promotes expansionary policies for the healthcare sector.

Similarly, Navarro et al. (2006) provides some nuanced evidence of an 'ideological effect' on health system reform. Countries governed by political parties of 'egalitarian views' have tended to implement redistributive policies in contrast to Christian-democratic (conservative), liberal, conservative-authoritarian (dictatorships). Navarro et al. (2006), examining the influence of parties' pro-redistributive nature, only find an association with lower infant mortality, but the effect was only significant for the sample of the 1990s and not for previous samples. The effect disappeared when other measures of health, such as life expectancy, were accounted for. Similarly, Mackenbach and McKee (2013) find that, indeed, ideology can be linked to public health policy. However, part of such effects might be time and country specific around politics of extending coverage. In addition, Potrafke (2010) shows that leftist governments increased overall social spending up to the end of the 1980s; but this partisan effect disappeared in the 1990s. In contrast, Schmidt (1999) discusses the lesser influence of government ideology on health. Specifically, explanations include its technical nature as well as certain middle-class and regulatory capture. The specific aspects of the health system that can be made electorally competitive are limited to healthcare coverage and aspects related to waiting lists when they are measurable. However, frequently, quality of care is highly unobservable and hence political ideologies are not constructed around it. Finally, a recent empirical study examining the effect of austerity policies in the area of healthcare (Reeves et al., 2014) shows that the ideology of governing parties had no effect on changes to healthcare spending. Instead, the authors find that countries which borrowed from the International Monetary Fund (IMF) were also less likely to protect healthcare budgets when they decided to implement austerity measures.

BELIEFS AND THE DEMAND SIDE

Theoretical and empirical models are able to match only partially demand and supply of policies. If supply is relatively easy to discuss with traditional categories like left and right party politics, socialist and liberal, the demand side is much less so. This is because it is unclear what makes the PC a liberal or a socialist, or any other ideology for the sake of the argument. This is an intriguing issue in understanding political processes in different countries. Of course, the supply side is important: the supply of ideologically oriented political platforms can influence voter turnout and adhesion to these platforms by the PC. In the case of healthcare, however, there are two approaches that get mixed up in the preference towards public healthcare. One approach conceptualises public healthcare as a redistributive mechanism. According to this view, public healthcare is useful as a tool for redistributing resources towards the poor; one would observe limited access to services if these were supplied only via private markets. This is clearly a view supported by left-wing parties, and likeminded people will be more likely to ideologically support left-leaning platforms. An alternative view conceives public healthcare as an insurance mechanism. According to this view public healthcare will serve as an insurance tool for all those unlucky to be sick. This is not necessarily a position supported by left-wing parties. Instead, liberals, in the continental European sense, are willing to extend public insurance against the risk of ill health.

The core of this debate prompts a discussion on the role of luck in determining economic outcomes, which has been shown to be an important driver of the demand for redistribution according to the analysis by Alesina et al. (2001). The crucial explanation is related to individual beliefs about what determines the place each one of us occupies in society. Understanding beliefs is important since they offer a representation of what people think; and they should be the direct determinant of their voting behaviour. To explore this issue, Alesina et al. (2001) consider data from the World Value Survey produced by the Institute for Social Research at the University of Michigan. The variables they focus on are responses to the following questions: the first, 'Why, in your opinion, are there people in this country who live in need? Here are two opinions: which comes closest to your view? They are poor because society treats them unfairly. They are poor because of laziness and lack will of power'; second, 'In your opinion, do most poor people in this country have a chance of escaping from poverty, or is there very little chance of escaping? They have a chance. There is very little chance.' A final question asks respondents to indicate agreement or disagreement with respect to the following statements: 'In the long run, hard work usually brings better life' and 'Hard work does not generally bring success, it is more a matter of luck and connections'. People that view luck as more important than effort will likely share the view that poor people are so because society treats them unfairly, and there is very little chance for them to escape from poverty. They will also likely disagree with the statement that hard work brings about a better life, and agree with the opposite statement that success is more a matter of luck and connections.

How different will a vote be of an individual who believes that luck is more important than effort? Alesina et al. (2001) show that these individuals are more likely to support political parties favouring redistribution, which tend to be, left-wing parties. These authors find a positive association between a leftist political orientation and the belief that luck determines income, controlling for income, gender, ethnicity, marital status, presence of children in the family. They also find a positive correlation between social spending (as percentage of GDP), including healthcare spending, and beliefs that luck determines income. This is unsurprising: as long as one thinks that luck is important, it is reasonable to demand further pro-poor redistribution, which then translates into a higher demand for social spending, expressed as a vote for left-wing parties. Interestingly, according to World Values Survey data, there are large differences between European countries and the United States in terms of beliefs, which explain the variations we observe in the approach towards the organisation of social protection and healthcare systems. In particular, 60 per cent of European citizens believe that the poor are trapped in poverty, against a share of 29 per cent of US citizens. Accordingly, 54 per cent of Europeans against 30 per cent of US residents believe that luck determines income. On the contrary, 60 per cent of US citizens believe that the poor are lazy against 26 per cent of European citizens. The fact that European beliefs are more oriented towards the role of luck is helpful in explaining their demand for redistribution, and for a larger spending in healthcare.

The idea that income, and hence the capacity to finance protection against healthcare risks, is either primarily determined by luck or primarily determined by effort is fundamental to explaining political ideologies that then translate into votes for political parties supporting these ideologies. However, this is certainly not the only idea that matters in explaining voters' behaviour towards the expansion of the public domain in healthcare. Alesina et al. (2001) discuss, for instance, the role of racial fractionalisation, which is defined according to the probability that a random selection of two individuals ends up with the two individuals being of a different race. Hence, racially fragmented societies are those where many different ethnicities coexist. In this sense, the United States or Brazil are more fractionalised than most of the European countries. Importantly, the authors show that there exists a negative correlation between racial fragmentation and social spending as a percentage of GDP. One likely explanation is that people indulge more towards redistribution in favour of the same kin. They prefer not to pay taxes if they know that revenues might be used by government to help fellow citizens that are of a different ethnic group.

This result is in line with what we are observing in the present day in more affluent societies, towards which the vast majority of migrants' flows are directed. Populist parties have emerged in most countries experiencing large migration inflows. For instance, findings by Dustmann et al. (2019) suggest that the vote shares of parties with an anti-immigration agenda (but also of centre-right parties) have increased in Denmark following a large inflow of refugee immigrants. Only large urban contexts seem to be unaffected. Importantly, voters' responses are different with respect to the degree to which existing immigrant populations are welfare dependent: higher dependency rates will lead to a stronger shift of votes to the anti-immigration parties as a result of refugee allocation. This type of political outcome will largely affect healthcare policies as well. One might expect that political support towards public healthcare policies will decrease as well if people believe that larger immigration flows, and hence a more ethnically fractionalised society, will be conducive to more consumption by someone who is not of the same kin.

THE ROLE OF THE MEDIA

The media are important stakeholders with respect to health and healthcare. DellaVigna and Kaplan (2007) found that in the USA, entry of Fox News into cable TV markets increased support of the Republican Party by 0.4–0.7 percentage points. There are at least three possible avenues through which the media can affect the demand for policies: first, the media can directly influence health by modifying individual behaviours; second, the media can shape individuals' beliefs by modifying perceptions about the role of luck and effort; third, the media can shape beliefs about how decision-makers in office or doctors work. Next, we discuss each of these possible channels.

The Media and Individual Behaviour

The media can affect individual behaviour in many different, and sometimes unexpected, ways. Educational programmes, supporting healthy lifestyles or showing the problems that excessive consumption of alcohol and drugs can have on health, can be used to promote health and prevent illnesses. However, the media can go an extra mile. For instance, La Ferrara et al. (2012) show that, in Brazil, soap operas broadcast on TV might be able to influence the reproductive behaviour of women. They can do so by portraying smaller families than those common in Brazil. The authors exploit differences in the timing of entry into different markets of Globo, the main 'novela' producer, and show that women living in areas covered by Globo have significantly lower fertility. The decline in the number of children is stronger for women of lower socio-economic status and for women in the central and late phases of fertility. In addition, the authors support the view that soap operas are driving the results, and not just television, since children's naming patterns follow 'novela' content. Clearly enough, if 'novelas' are able to influence reproductive behaviour, commercial movies showing unhealthy behaviours like binge drinking or drugs consumption will likely have similar effects. As an example, Gutschoven and Van den Bulck (2004) show that television viewing is significantly related to the number of cigarettes smoked. One explanation is that its portrayal on television may make smoking attractive, inducing more children to start smoking in a similar way as 'novelas' make small families more attractive, inducing more women to reduce the number of children they give birth to.

The Media and Beliefs about Role of Luck and Effort

The media can alter perceptions and beliefs of PCs with respect to the role of luck and effort in determining income in a number of different ways. For instance, commercial, easy-to-consume television can shape ideals and make people vote more for populist parties, an effect documented in Durante et al. (2018) exploiting the introduction of commercial TV by Mr Berlusconi in Italy. The media can make people more or less pessimistic about intergenerational mobility and this change in beliefs will increase or decrease support for redistributive policies. A randomised survey experiment reported in Alesina et al. (2018), conducted in France, Italy, Sweden, the UK and the USA, supports the view that information making people more pessimistic about social mobility increases support for 'equality of opportunity' policies.

The Media and Health System Beliefs

The role of the media in informing PCs can have large effects shaping beliefs on how politicians and doctors involved in the management of the system work. As an example, Le Moglie and Turati (2019) show the existence of an 'electoral cycle bias' in the coverage of corruption news relative to the Italian regional healthcare system by two of the most important national newspapers, which are also characterised by a clear ideological stance, namely *La Repubblica* (left-wing oriented) and *Il Giornale* (right-wing oriented). The Italian NHS is a regional system; hence, corruption news is highly salient for regional elections. The authors find that news outlets' ideologies influence the reporting of corruption news when regional elections approach. The strategy adopted by the two newspapers is similar and suggests that the media increases the number of articles about differently minded politicians, while reducing the amount of those that address episodes of corruption without any political connection. While the authors are unable to connect this finding to electoral outcomes because of the reduced quantity of observations available, they discuss anecdotal evidence showing that corruption news led to the resignation of an important regional president of Lombardy, Mr Formigoni, and to a significant drop in the vote share of the right-wing coalition.

Another example is the work by Sangrigoli et al. (2018), which analyses two cases of corruption in a large Italian hospital, involving the CEO and a famous surgeon. The hospital CEO was caught receiving bribes in his office to favour a patient on the waiting list for a kidney transplant. The well-known heart surgeon in charge of the regional Heart Transplant Centre was accused of accepting large sums of money in exchange for the supply rights of cardiac valves from two specific firms. Media reporting about corruption not only influences the beliefs of the PC, but also those of people working within the healthcare system, who take up both the role of the PC and the role of colleagues of those involved in the corruption scandal. The authors show that corruption news had sizeable effects in terms of the reduction of the number of potential donors reported to the coordination centre.

A similar effect is documented when television programmes aim at informing PCs about physicians' behaviour. A very famous case was 'Panorama', a BBC TV broadcast in 1980. The programme raised doubts on the issue of brain death, which differentiates legal death from biological death. A brain-dead patient is one that has completely lost brain function. The definition developed from a

1968 report signed by a committee at Harvard Medical School and it is well established in laws and regulation around the world. Ascertaining whether a patient is brain-dead is preliminary to organ retrieval. The BBC programme questioned doctors' professional standards in defining brain-dead patients. Unsurprisingly, this made people cautious about doctors and dramatically reduced organ donations, an effect that lasted for over a year (Matesanz, 1996).

THE POLITICAL CYCLE AND HEALTHCARE

Healthcare decision-making is frequently argued to be 'politicised', which implies that the political cycle does indeed play a role in influencing policymaking. Some important research has been carried out to examine the political cycle in healthcare, which differentiates standard ideological decision-making from pure electoral interests, namely opportunism. Potrafke (2010) finds evidence of opportunism in healthcare policymaking rather than ideology. Opportunistic policy makers can fool the naive PC, especially when they can exploit an informational advantage on quality, as in the healthcare area. In such a case, one can make salient political health decisions, such as approving regulation that expands healthcare coverage shortly before an election to gain political support. However, the latter might not be true when decision-making entails conflicting choices in the context of austerity, as there are limited opportunities for political incumbents to claim credit in such contexts.

The capacity for politicians to strategically increase spending before an election is affected by the individual specific characteristics of political incumbents (Potrafke, 2010). Male and female politicians display different ideas with respect to health. For instance, Bhalotra and Clots-Figueras (2014) investigate whether women's political representation improves public provision of antenatal and childhood health services in the districts from which they are elected. In Indian states, as in most developing and developed countries, the costs of poor maternal and childhood healthcare services fall disproportionately upon women. The authors find that an increase in women's representation implies a reduction in neonatal mortality. The mechanisms behind this result seems to be driven by differing approaches from male and female politicians with respect to infrastructures supplied to local communities. Male politicians seem to be more oriented towards supplying financial and telecommunications infrastructures, while female politicians are more likely to invest in healthcare facilities. This facilitates the reduction in home births, generally unattended by medical professionals, and the increase of deliveries in government facilities. According to the authors of the study, these results support the view that women's political representation may be a tool for addressing healthcare needs in developing countries.

Other potential characteristics can include the specific professional background and training of political incumbents. When medical doctors take up political offices they might take advantage of their prior knowledge of the health system, but their actions could be constrained by the specific medical association they are regulated by, and can be subject to regulatory capture and lobby by their own peers (Coretti et al., 2020).

Previous job experience and professional affiliation play a role. In the context of healthcare, Francese et al. (2014) study the role of politicians' characteristics, in particular those of regional presidents on the share of C-sections in Italian regions. The authors find that experienced politicians are better able to manage resources and increase appropriateness. In other words, politicians that have been in office for longer periods obtain better results in terms of providing appropriate care. This effect turns positive if the incumbent president is aligned with the central government, in other words they are supported by the same political parties or coalition. A possible interpretation is that one can always expect a favourable treatment by an ideologically close government, so experience is less important. An additional interesting finding is that occupation before entering politics does matter. In particular, being a physician is associated with an increase in inappropriateness and inefficiency, most likely because physicians are subject to regulatory capture, are prone to lobbying from their colleagues and implement a weaker regulation. A similar result is provided in Pilny and Roesel (2017), who exploit data on German state health ministers. These ministers enjoy great autonomy in defining hospital policies. The authors find that total factor productivity growth slows down when physicians become health ministers. This is due to the fact that they increase employment of their colleagues while leaving hospital outputs unchanged.

SUMMARY

This chapter has examined the role of ideologies and ideas more generally in the formation of health policies. We have examined how left-wing and right-wing parties represent their electorate's healthcare policies. Right-wing parties tend to be associated with key concepts like competition, markets and the proliferation of private providers. In contrast, left-wing parties tend to have in mind some level of public funding, as well as a redistributive view of public healthcare towards the low and middle class.

We then discussed the role of individual beliefs in shaping the demand for redistribution on the PC side. We showed the importance of luck and effort as drivers for individual income as key determinants of the demand for redistribution, a demand which also fuels the demand for more public spending in healthcare. We also discussed the role of ethnic fractionalisation, showing that in more racially fragmented societies, the demand for redistribution is lower. We dedicated a section to the role of the media in influencing individual behaviour and in shaping individual beliefs. Finally, we suggested that politicians can try to influence voters by strategically using healthcare spending among other spending categories. This brings us to the idea that the characteristics of incumbent politicians, such as their experience, professional background and gender, matter. Although old data suggests evidence of a strong ideological effect, such ideological influences have disappeared in the context of the recent austerity period.

PART IV Political Allocation in Healthcare

8   Healthcare Waste and Corruption

Ernest A. Codman, a surgeon at Massachusetts General Hospital, proposed back in 1910 that each hospital should track every patient to determine whether the treatment the hospital provided was effective (McIntyre et al., 2001). This 'end result system of hospital standardization' proposed by Codman was one of the first systematic attempts to assess the performance of healthcare activity. In modern terms, Codman's idea was to understand the extent to which monies were spent on high-value care instead of low-value treatments. To his surprise, the assessment of resource allocation was not an activity that was particularly appreciated by hospital managers, given that it made their actions more transparent, which in turn reduced the room for opportunistic behaviours of different kinds, including waste (and corruption). As Codman puts it, 'our charitable hospitals do not consider it their duty to see that good results are obtained in the treatment of their patients... It is against the individual interests of the medical and surgical staffs of hospitals to follow up, compare, analyze, and standardize all their results' because (i) 'perhaps the results as a whole would not be good enough to impress the public very favorably'; (ii) it is 'difficult, time-consuming, and troublesome'; and (iii) 'neither the hospital trustees nor the public are as yet willing to pay for this kind of work' (McIntyre et al., 2001, p. 9). Codman was clear in identifying the conflict of interest for medical and surgical performance measurement. But it is not only the medical or the surgical staff involved that he thought would be exposed. In publicly funded systems, politicians in charge of funding or regulating health care have more room to manoeuvre the less transparent healthcare practices are, or the harder it becomes for the general public to have access to performance information and subject the hospitals to closer connections between spending and performance.

In this chapter we begin by discussing how modern healthcare systems waste resources. We then review some empirical evidence identifying which systems are less efficient, and then focus on corruption, a particularly disreputable part of the inefficiency plaguing the industry. Broadly speaking, health systems are subject to two major sources of waste. One type includes what we could describe as 'market source', and especially refers to the types of waste related to plain over-consumption as well as overtreatment, inappropriate prescriptions, mis-diagnosis, coordination failures and organisational slack (known as x-inefficiency), which affect both the management and the bureaucratic nature of healthcare organisations. Common to these phenomena is that they can occur without corruption or illegitimate and illegal activity.

The second source of waste is commonly known as corruption, which in the healthcare sector mostly refers to bureaucratic corruption. Bribes or a higher price granted arbitrarily, to a company are examples of 'waste', since they usually imply agreements that entail that the patient citizen (PC) ends up paying prices above the standard rate, including deadweight losses associated with extra taxation. However, as Acemoglu and Verdier (1998) argue, this might be a 'necessary evil', as public involvement might come with some corruption, but also solves market failures. That is, thicker profits and bureaucrats' salaries come at the expense of the wellbeing of the PC, in terms of lower quality and higher cost of care. In such a setting, a scenario of no public healthcare at all to fully avoid corruption of public officials might be worse than public healthcare of lower quality than optimal, and with some (inevitable) corruption. Hence, a cold-hearted reading of such an argument would indicate that welfare losses from corruption might be a 'necessary evil', though they entail an unfair and illegitimate redistribution. Yet, it poses a threat to the functioning, and more generally the support of the health system by the PC, which might see a corrupt system as suffering from a 'leaky bucket' (Okun, 1975), which is accepted depending on its size (e,g. higher corrpution might incentivise the opting out to using private health care alternatives).

In the presence of corruption, it is important to point out that there are winners and losers from corrupt activities. Hence if one wants to make an assessment, interpersonal comparisons of utility are inescapable. Is one dollar to a corrupt bureaucrat worth less than one dollar more to the PC from a welfare point of view? Second, given that corruption exposes those engaging in such activity to the risk of being caught, then part of their activities emerge as efforts to be stealthy, which would otherwise not be needed in a legal tax environment (Shleifer and Vishny, 1993), and give rise to thus net efficiency losses. The effort to reduce the uncertainty of being caught and cover this behaviour is thus a pure waste. Third, corruption can be systemic and lead to diffused uncertainty about what rules are to be followed. This is because when *de jure* and de facto bounds about what is permitted by law become blurry and more so as corruption becomes pervasive (Shleifer and Vishny, 1993).

EXPLAINING 'RED TAPE'

Waste or Inefficiency?

The US healthcare system is clearly the costliest at the international level: in absolute terms, per capita average spending in the USA amounted to $10,348 in 2016, 425 times the spending of a very poor sub-Saharan country like Zimbabwe (where spending amounted to $24.34 according to data provided by UNICEF). Despite such levels of investment, the US population is not the healthiest in the world. Average life expectancy at birth in the USA, about seventy-eight years, is clearly above that of Zimbabwe, which is about sixty years. But, for instance, it is below that of the UK by about three years on average, with the UK spending substantially less than the USA. This prompts the question: what factors explain such differences in productivity?

The view of an economist of how (public and private) resources are translated into health outcomes helps identifying what we mean by waste: healthcare systems are said to be inefficient if they waste scarce resources which can be 'better invested'. If other countries are attaining better outcomes than the USA with the same level of investment one could argue that the US system is 'relatively' more inefficient. This, of course, is not totally accurate as one would need to adjust outcomes by measures of quality prices, and possibly isolate health expenditures that are influencing other non-health aspects of the health system. However, on aggregate it appears that one could attain the same outcomes with less investment by adopting other healthcare organisations. Hence, although more investment might make a difference, it seems clear that the institutional design of the health system can help in reducing waste.

There are, by now, many scholars suggesting that the best strategy to improve the health of US citizens should start with reducing waste in order to obtain better health by spending less (e.g. Garber and Skinner, 2008). Berwick and Hackbarth (2012) provide a detailed computation of the amount of resources that can be recovered by eliminating waste together with a taxonomy of waste categories (which is important to start thinking about in order to determine how we can tackle wasteful spending). More specifically, Table 8.1 shows the total costs of waste in the USA. According to the most conservative estimates, total waste in 2011 amounted to $197 billion for Medicare and Medicaid only. Considering the US healthcare system as a whole, these costs rise to $558 billion, which amounts to 21 per cent of total spending. The importance of considering waste is more than obvious when numbers involved are as large as those represented here.

Overtreatment

Table 8.1 depicts estimates of the most common sources of healthcare waste in the United States. It shows that the most significant category

Table 8.1 *Estimates of annual US healthcare waste*[a]

	\$ billions					
	Annual cost to Medicare and Medicaid in 2011[b]			Annual cost to US healthcare system in 2011		
	Low	Midpoint	High	Low	Midpoint	High
Failures of care delivery	26	36	45	102	128	154
Failures of care coordination	21	30	39	25	35	45
Overtreatment	67	77	87	158	192	226
Administrative complexity	16	36	56	107	248	389
Pricing failures	36	56	77	84	131	178
Fraud and abuse	30	64	98	82	177	272
Total[c]	**197**	**300**	**402**	**558**	**910**	**1,263**
% of total spending				**21**	**34**	**47**

Notes: [a] Table entries represent the range of estimates of waste in each category from sources cited in the text. The total waste estimates are simply the sums of the category-level estimates. This simple summing is feasible because the categories are defined in such a way that wasteful behaviours could be assigned to at most one category and because, like Pacala and Socolow, we did not attempt to estimate interactions between or among the categories.
[b] Including both state and federal costs.
[c] Totals may not match the sum of components due to rounding.
Source: Berwick and Hackbarth (2012)

of waste refers to *overtreatment*. Overtreatment entails subjecting patients to care that – according to medical knowledge, and even considering patient preferences – cannot help them. Examples include excessive use of antibiotics, use of surgery when watchful waiting (vs, e.g. radical prostatectomy in early prostate cancer) or unwanted intensive care at the end of life when patients simply prefer home care (Brownlee et al., 2017). In a number of cases, overtreatment refers to inappropriate treatment. A treatment is inappropriate when care can be delivered in a cheaper and safer way, or when it does not follow clinical guidelines. Overtreatment includes over-medicalisation, in other words the excessive use in richer and advanced societies of medical and surgical treatments when they are not needed (Conrad, 2007). Different clinical practices in obstetrics provide a clear way to think about over-medicalisation. In some countries, such as the Netherlands, we can observe an increasing number of women giving birth at home. At the end of the spectrum of this over-medicalisation lies C-sections, a surgical procedure. There has been an overall global trend towards an increase in the share of C-sections out of the total number of deliveries. This is not to say that all C-sections are inappropriate and not needed: reproductive behaviour has changed, especially in some Western countries, with total fertility rates plummeting and the age of the mother at first delivery rising steadily over time. Older mothers would likely run a higher risk of incurring a C-section for medical reasons. However, this is just part of the story. Economists refer to the impact of a better organisation of working shifts in the case of elective C-sections as well as the role of financial incentives, as C-sections are better reimbursed than vaginal deliveries; hence, there is a financial incentive for hospitals that – in the absence of a well-implemented audit programme – is reflected in a higher probability for physicians to choose a C-section, even when it is inappropriate (Mossialos et al., 2005). Other examples include common practice of 'upcoding' patients' diagnostic-related groups (DRGs) to increase the reimbursement hospitals obtain from insurers (Silverman and Skinner, 2004).

Administrative Complexity

Waste can also result from *administrative complexity*. In this case, it is caused by inefficient or misguided institutions, such as rules dictated by government agencies or third-party payers which fail to serve the purpose of such organisations. For instance, rules that make physicians spend their limited time on administrative duties instead of devoting their care to patients. On the patient end, complexity is reflected in procedures that limit the patient capacity to navigate the health system and follow rules to obtain the treatments. Problems of complexity take a toll on healthcare costs in a highly fragmented markets (Cutler et al., 2012). For instance, Casalino et al. (2009) calculate that the average US physician spends 43 minutes per day discussing with different health insurance plans to obtain authorisations for procedures and payments instead of devoting more time to patients. However, the increase in administrative tasks for physicians is also a source of concern in mostly public healthcare systems.

Failures of Care Delivery

Waste might not only be the result of limited design, but *poor treatment execution* as well as lack of widespread adoption of the most effective treatments, including preventive care and patient safety systems. For instance, Skinner and Staiger (2015) study three fundamental innovations in the treatment of acute myocardial infarction (AMI) which developed during the 1990s: first, aspirin, which improves blood flow to oxygen-starved tissue and has been included in US standard guidelines for care since 1988; second, a beta-blocker, an inexpensive drug; third, the reperfusion of the heart muscles within twelve hours of the AMI using either thrombolytics drugs or a percutaneous coronary intervention (PCI). Not all hospitals adopt the most effective technologies to treat AMI. The average gap in survival between patients hospitalised in the slowest adopter hospitals and the quickest adopters is on average 2.7 percentage points, which clearly shows the importance of waste reduction as well as the potential for health improvement of the PC.

Pricing Failures

A fourth cause of waste, in terms of resources dissipated, is the one related with *pricing failures*, which generally refers to large rents available for producers of services, as well as for suppliers and insurers when prices are far from competitive. That is, when prices exceed the marginal costs of production plus a fair profit. Among the reasons for pricing failures lies the fact that producers of health services enjoy market power, either *ex ante* because of them being local monopolists, or *ex post* because of the lock-in contracts that arise when a patient patronises a given provider. For example, Berwick and Hackbarth (2012) find that US prices for diagnostic procedures like magnetic resonance imaging and computerised tomography scans are several times those reported in other countries for similar procedures. Hsia et al. (2014) reported marked variation across Californian hospitals for charges related to vaginal deliveries and C-sections. As for the former, the observed range was \$3,344–\$43,715; for the latter \$7,905–\$72,569. The problem is also particularly severe in the case of newly developed drugs that enjoy patent protection. Another pathway to pricing failures arises when prices are regulated and sometimes used to provide incentives or disincentives to healthcare producers. In the latter case, pricing failures result from regulation failures, which we will discuss in detail in Chapter 9. In some specific cases one can also argue that private producers capture regulators and lobby them to obtain better pricing conditions (see, e.g. the evidence provided in Francese et al., 2014, for C-sections tariffs in Italy).

Fraud and Corruption

One of the most important categories of waste according to patients' *self-reported perceptions is fraud*. Paradoxically, according to most estimates around the world, waste from corruption is just a small fraction of inefficient spending in healthcare. For instance, Bandiera et al. (2009) examined the purchases of standardised goods by Italian public bodies and find that some public bodies pay systematically more than others for equivalent goods. The authors try then to provide an explanation of the observed variation in prices distinguishing between two types of waste: 'passive' waste (which they define according to organisational or x-inefficiencies and limited work incentive) and 'active' waste (which mainly refers to corruption). They find that price variation is mainly due to passive rather than active waste. In particular, active waste explains just 17 per cent of total estimated waste. However, individual perceptions about the prevalence of corruption are driven by the fact that fraud requires an active role by the staff looking for personal advantages. Examples include fake bills to justify payments or absenteeism of medical staff. We will provide a detailed analysis of this category of waste below.

Coordination Failures

Finally, some resources are wasted because of *failures in care coordination*. For instance, care coordination among different providers is required for the treatment of chronic patients, a category of patients increasing in numbers in recent decades. Waste arises because of the fragmented nature of the health system, which eventually produces extra complications, hospital readmissions, functional status decline, increased dependency and higher costs. For instance, Frandsen et al. (2015) show that a more fragmented style of practice in the USA has resulted in a greater number of primary care visits, as well as more specialists' visits.

Of course, by being the top-spending country, the USA is the most striking example of the presence of absolute waste in healthcare expenditure. However, other countries might exhibit a higher level of relative waste (to GDP or health expenditure). At some level, all healthcare systems waste resources due to coordination failures. According to numbers provided by the Organisation for Economic Co-operation and Development (OECD), nearly one-third of total health expenditure in Australia could be deemed wasteful; similarly, 20 per cent of the budget for acute care could be saved by reducing overutilisation and increasing integration of care in the Netherlands

(Couffinhal and Socha-Dietrich, 2017). This is especially concerning in publicly funded systems, since waste is inextricably related to the departure from competitive markets which characterise the markets of healthcare delivery of services, the supply of medical devices and healthcare insurance. Hence, part of health system design is to reduce the amount of waste rather than to eliminate it completely.

There are a number of exercises in the literature studying the efficiency of different healthcare systems. Some of these exercises have made newspaper headlines: they are simple to understand, and they report a clear ranking of countries that journalists love to use. The ranking of countries estimated by Bloomberg[1] provides one such example: it compares healthcare spending relative to GDP (resources) with life expectancy at birth (outcome). Singapore and Hong Kong stand out among the best performers since life expectancy is as high as eighty-three years, while spending is relatively low (about 5 per cent of GDP). A similar argument can be made for the Italian and the Spanish healthcare systems within Europe. The USA is in the fiftieth position, below countries like Algeria, where life expectancy is a bit lower than in the USA (seventy-four years vs seventy-eight years) but spending is much lower (in per capita terms, $362 vs $9,403, 2014 data).

A different example is provided by the 2000 World Health Report (World Health Organization (WHO), 2000), which considers five main variables to assess the performance of different countries: the overall level of health (measured by Disability Adjusted Life Expectancy); the distribution of health in the population; the overall level of responsiveness (measured with a survey trying to understand how the system meets patients' expectations of how they should be treated by providers); the distribution of responsiveness; and the

---

[1] http://largest-biggest.com/index.php/2017/05/15/bloomberg-most-efficient-health-care-systems-in-the-world/ (last accessed 18 August 2018).

distribution of financial contribution. The overall attainment of a system is a combination of these five indicators and has to be compared with the level of resources that has been consumed by the country (healthcare spending). Results show that even adjusting for disability and considering responsiveness, Singapore, Italy and Spain (Hong Kong not considered here) rank in the top ten positions. However, the USA (thirty-seventh) is only above Algeria (eighty-first) since correction for disability matters greatly and the Algerian system is much less responsive than that of the USA, likely because of corruption problems (perceptions of corruption suggesting that this is an issue in the country; see Transparency International, 2006). Zimbabwe is 155th out of 191 countries in the WHO ranking: its system contributes poorly to health, it is very unresponsive and it is very financially unfair, so that despite spending less than the Abuja target of 15 per cent of GDP, the performance is very poor. Unlike the Bloomberg exercise, controversy about the results published in the report was high, as reported in Veillard et al. (2009): critics looked at the scarce attention to primary care as well as the coherence of performance measures, the validity of rankings and the use of estimates instead of actual data. Controversy, however, is not surprising since – as we have already noted – publication of benchmarking exercises improves transparency and asks those managing the system to provide an answer to the assessment they received. If waste is inextricably linked to healthcare systems all around the world, then we need to learn more about it, starting with how we can assess it.

SOURCES OF INEFFICIENCIES AND MEASUREMENT

A possible central way to help reduce waste in a health system lies in its measurement and identification. For the PC to form its Wicksellian connections around different health policies, one would need to be able to identify how much waste exists in today's healthcare systems. The measurement of waste is one of those policy interventions on which almost all stakeholders, namely insurers, PCs and possibly providers, are on the same page, except providers that benefit from it, namely the medical device and pharmaceutical industries. Overtreatment increases the revenues of such companies, and hence are not incentivised to spot the best clinical practices.

One way to identify inefficiency at the aggregate level is to compare the evidence on different OECD healthcare systems around the world. One could compare representative countries, considering input measures (per capita spending, physical inputs like number of hospital beds), outcome measures (life expectancy at birth, infant mortality, self-perceived health) and output measures (number of inpatient days, pharmaceutical spending). Such analysis would entail examining simple efficiency indicators by looking at a measure of health outcomes and comparing it to the investment per capita, which leads us to the Bloomberg example. However, in such a setting, a point can be made that such indicators are incomplete, which takes us to the World Health Report containing a specific index weighting different measures of health system outcomes. A more refined approach might consider estimating a production/cost frontier, using Data Envelopment Analysis or other econometric techniques discussed in, for example, Kumbhakar and Knox Lovell, 2000; Fried et al., 2007; and Hollingsworth and Peacock, 2008. Finally, one could consider the role of changes over time as in Skinner and Staiger (2015) and discuss the role of technological innovation alongside different diffusion production functions for varied technologies (discussed in Chapter 10).

However, even when inefficiencies are measured, it is possible to claim that inefficiencies stem from organisational choices at different levels, which include a number of institutional variables affecting the health system, such as the level of governance (e.g. decentralise the health system or not), the specific mission of payers (e.g. public or private insurance) and providers (public or private producers, quasi-markets or integrated models, non-profit or for-profit private providers) and, of course, the various agency relationships at different levels opening up room for opportunistic behaviour.

CHARACTERISING CORRUPTION

As discussed above, fraud is just one type of inefficiency, and not even the most important one in quantitative terms. According to Aidt (2003, p. F632), corruption is 'an act in which the power of public office is used for personal gain in a manner that contravenes the rules of the game'. Similarly, Vian (2008, p. 84) argues that 'corruption occurs when public officials who have been given the authority to carry out goals which further the public good, instead use their position and power to benefit themselves and others close to them'. In both cases, corruption entails a public official who has power and uses it for personal gains to the detriment of society. However, it is precisely the fact that corruption results from a deliberate action by healthcare stakeholders that makes it more unacceptable and, possibly, unethical. However, as we have claimed, it is the institutional design of the health system that opens the door to opportunistic behaviour.

Figure 8.1 describes the potential avenues for corruption that can emerge in practice. Consider the key actors defining the healthcare system: regulators, payers, healthcare providers, patients and suppliers of medical equipments and drugs. As we have already discussed, many of these actors represent broad categories that can include many different institutions or are aligned with the political choices made in a country. Public regulators, the first of these actors, can be represented, for instance, by the Ministry of Health, the national parliament or some other governmental agency in centralised healthcare systems, but also by regional parliaments or municipality boards in countries where healthcare regulation has been decentralised at the local level. Furthermore, the Ministry of Health or some national agencies might be responsible for fixing the prices of

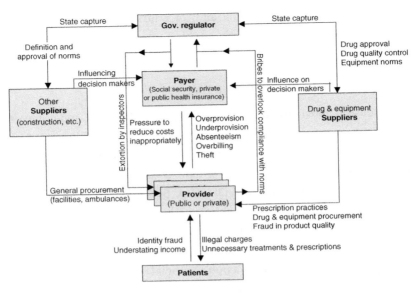

FIGURE 8.1 The net of corruption in healthcare systems
Source: Savedoff and Hussman (2006)

drugs, while regional or local governments are responsible for regulating the quasi-market for hospital services. As for corruption, all of
these regulators can be captured in different ways by other institutions (particularly suppliers and producers) working within the
system: striking examples include, on the one hand, powerful pharmaceutical companies that influence review boards or bribe regulators to
have a swifter approval of their applications, and on the other hand
hospitals or other producers of health services that pay regulators in
order to overlook lapses in licensing requirements or to obtain better
payments for their supply. As an example, consider the case of
Schering-Plough Poland– Chudow Castle Foundation reported in the
Global Corruption Report 2006. The Polish subsidiary of the US-based
pharmaceutical company made payments to a foundation for the
restoration of Silesian castles. According to allegations by the US
Security and Exchange Commission, which fined the company for
violations of the books and records and internal controls provisions
of the Foreign Corrupt Practices Act (FCPA), the foundation was run

by the director of the Silesian Health Fund, one of the local regulators in the public Polish healthcare system. Almost all the defining features of corruption were present here: a public official (the director of the Silesian Fund), who had the power to decide whether to buy a given drug and accept a payment (the personal gain). However, on the other side, public officials can also be tempted to bribe private firms (either pharmaceutical firms or hospitals) even if they are compliant.

A second key actor is represented by payers. Payers vary widely across different countries. The public sector can act as a player in publicly, funded healthcare systems, either funding the provision of care directly, or acting as a public insurer. In this case, corruption can emerge as a result of payers searching for political gains instead of patients' interests. For instance, regulators can partly divert funds to regional governments that are politically aligned instead of focusing more on patients' needs. Evidence supporting this 'alignment effect', typical in decentralised systems with vertical relationships between layers of governments, have been found in countries as different as India, Germany, Italy and the USA, to name a few (Besley and Case, 2003; Arulampalam et al., 2009; Bordignon and Turati, 2009; Baskaran and Hessami, 2017; Kleider et al., 2018). On the other hand, in privately funded systems, payers are represented either by private for-profit insurance companies supplying coverage together with non-profit or cooperative organisations, or patients paying out-of-pocket for the services they need. In this case, private insurers can defraud public sector programmes subsidising coverage, like in the USA, via false charges, bribing regulators to ignore illegal behaviour.

Healthcare providers are, of course, at the centre of corrupt activities, since these actors are the ones making most of the relevant medical decisions. There is a wide range of providers, in terms of both ownership structure (from public to private non-profit and for-profit) and services involved (primary care, hospitals, long-term care). In all cases, patients refer to medical staff to navigate the system, and understand what service 'to buy', and this clearly creates substantial room for the staff to exercise discretionary power and the opportunities to take advantage of the PC. Different providers are characterised by various incentives and moral and ethical constraints: for instance, there is evidence in the literature that for-profit providers are those less ethically constrained (e.g. Horwitz, 2007), which can be explained by for-profit organisations being ethically less constrained by constitution. Examples of fraud and abuse in this case include physicians, also employed in public hospitals, referring patients to their private practice or even creating 'phantom' patients to obtain larger reimbursements from payers' staff, or stealing drugs and other supplies for resale. A very crude example is the case discussed in Holmberg and Rothstein (2011) of a mother in India who was asked for a bribe soon after giving birth to hold her child directly on her chest (the price was $12 for a boy, and $7 for a girl, a substantial amount of money in a country where the woman's husband was working for less than $1 per day).

Patients themselves can also participate in corruptive practices. For instance, they might try to get free care by under-reporting their income in systems where a co-payment is required to access some services, or they can pay bribes to gain access to services. In some countries, these bribes have become socially acceptable. For instance, in Greece there is a large black economy in the field of obstetric services (as documented by, e.g. Kaitelidou et al., 2013).

Finally, suppliers of drugs and equipments have privileged information on the quality of the products and services they sell, which helps them to introduce corruptive practices into the system. A very common example is that of suppliers bribing procurement officers or medical staff to sell their products better, for example by obtaining higher prices for products of lower value. As reported by Transparency International (2006), Germany investigated 450 hospitals and more than 2,700 doctors on suspicion of taking bribes from manufacturers of heart valves, life support equipment, cardiac pacemakers and hip joints. A similar case has been discovered in a large Italian hospital, creating a corruption scandal that will be discussed below.

Why are there so many avenues for corruption in the healthcare systems? The healthcare sector is more prone to corruption than other economic sectors because of its intrinsic characteristics. According to the discussion in Chapter 1, two problems emerge as crucial in the analysis by Arrow (1963): the presence of asymmetric information at various levels, between healthcare providers and the PCs, but also between producers of different services within the industry and between payers and providers. Asymmetric information generates a problem of trust at different levels, and opens the door to opportunistic behaviours given the discretionary power in the hands of the public official. The second characteristic is the presence of numerous conflicts of interest: situations in which the judgement by a health professional or a government official on a primary interest (the health of patients) conflicts with a secondary interest (a personal gain, not only in monetary terms). However, as noted by, for example Vian (2008), the joint occurrence of asymmetric information and conflicts of interest opens up opportunities for abuse (see Figure 8.2). This does not need to translate into actual abuse if – for instance – moral beliefs by an individual prevent them from abusing power. Consider the following real example: the management of a large hospital in Kenya realised that fees paid by citizens were stolen. This was a big issue, since about one-quarter of total hospital expenditures were covered by these fees. Moreover, patients complained about being bribed by staff at the hospital. Let us analyse this situation with the scheme provided by Figure 8.2: where does the room for abuse come from? The management realised that the system for collecting fees was designed to allow ample room for discretion: there was a highly decentralised system of collection within the hospital, manual receipts and infrequent audits, all of which clearly allowed room for opportunistic behaviour, and reduced transparency and accountability in favour of those cashing the fees. What about pressures to exploit? One might think that wages and salaries were low enough to introduce a strong pressure to exploit, however, not all the staff might have fallen prey to this, depending on ethical norms, personality traits or moral attitudes.

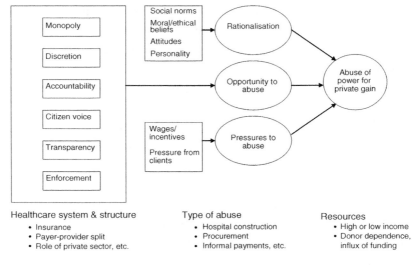

FIGURE 8.2 How corruption emerges
Source: Vian (2008)

Interestingly, to reduce corruption the management focused on reducing the opportunity for abuse: reducing the number of points for collecting fees, introducing electronic recording of fees and separating the billing procedure from the cashing procedure. This resulted in fees increasing by 47 per cent in the following three months, without any variation in the services provided.

WHAT ARE THE CONSEQUENCES OF CORRUPTION?

Corruption boosts expenditure, but the real scale of the problem is mostly difficult to estimate. Transparency International suggests that corruption amounts to tens of billions of dollars per year worldwide. However, this is just the easiest of the consequences to spot. The biggest issue is to understand the consequences on health, either directly or indirectly via the access to services or the reactions to corruption scandals. There are currently not many academic studies on this issue. One example is Azfar and Gurgur (2008) in the Philippines, where the healthcare system is decentralised at the local level given the geography of the country. The authors find that corruption reduces immunisation rates, delays the vaccination of newborns, reduces satisfaction with services and increases waiting times. As for the indirect consequences, the reporting corruption news by the media can undermine trust at different levels, both of patients and medical staff working within the system. Sangrigoli et al. (2018) provide an example by studying the reaction of the medical staff to two corruption scandals affecting one large public hospital in Italy. The first one was reported by the media in December 2001, when the hospital CEO was caught accepting bribes in his office and, after that, was charged with favouring a patient on a waiting list for a kidney. In November 2002 a second scandal occurred: a well-known heart surgeon was accused of favouring the use of specific cardiac valves supplied by two firms paying large sums of monies to the surgeon and one of his colleagues. The news made newspaper headlines at both the local and the national level. The study by Sangrigoli et al. (2018) provides evidence of the indirect effect of these two scandals on the procurement of organs in Piedmont. The econometric analysis shows that corruption lessens the number of organs via reduction in the number of reported donors. The authors interpret this finding as the emotional reaction of the medical staff when knowing that a colleague is corrupt, which crowds out the intrinsic motivation of the staff working in Intensive Care Units and reduces the effort to avoid organ deterioration.

SUMMARY

In this chapter, we have argued that healthcare systems are affected by inefficiencies and waste. This is, in part, the result of the joint occurrence of mismatch of incentives and asymmetric information, but can also result from ill-defined institutions, and in some cases end up in corruption. We have argued that some of the reasons for such waste and inefficiencies lie in a number of underpinning determinants such as payment systems that are open to opportunities for mismanagement and corruption, as well as organisation structures and limited coordination that benefit vested interests, such as the medical industry, as well as its limited transparency, and to an extent acceptance of the patient citizens and providers in the health system. The reduction of waste and corruption is fundamental for a health system to keep to its mission without running out of funds in a setting where there are limited resources available to invest in healthcare. This involves understanding the political design of the resource allocation within each health system to identify opportunities for a heavy influence by interest groups.

Overall, public intervention in healthcare is advocated in order to increase the welfare of the patient by granting access, through paying or directly supplying healthcare goods and services from a public programme or an overall national system. And it often does so. However, public intervention creates also the opportunity for waste and adds an additional layer of political agency, a misalignment of incentives plus asymmetric information, to the already complex entanglement of players' interactions that is classically present in healthcare. These two factors might create additional incentives for corruptive behaviour on the part of politicians, bureaucrats and stakeholders, which adds to that already present in the private sector.

9 Interest Groups and Health Policy

INTEREST GROUPS IN HEALTHCARE

In any health system there are stakeholders than have 'vested or special interests'. That is, that pursue a private gain (e.g. profit) as its main goal. When special interests run the health system, it runs the risk of departing from attaining its collective mission of improving the health and welfare of its population. This has led to a strand of the literature that examines the mechanisms that such interest groups use to attain their goals. This includes the design of the underpinning institutions in place in each health system.

This chapter discusses the role of some of the most striking examples of government failure, namely the influence of interest groups in health policymaking. Nonetheless, such actions might not necessarily be at odds with efficiency if such actions are conducive to socially beneficial decisions (Tullock, 1980). Interest groups are important demand-side actors, providing information, resources or political support to politicians (Grossman and Helpman, 2001). They influence policy by investing resources to steer decisions towards their private interests. Specifically, in this chapter we distinguish two different types of interest group activity, namely (i) the influence on healthcare regulation producing, and more specifically, the phenomenon of 'regulatory capture' and (ii) the competitive pursuit of a reallocation of healthcare budgets away from efficiency through rent-seeking.

The inefficiency of interest groups' influences in healthcare decision-making depends on how they compete to gain monopoly rents (from redirecting resources to new allocations by means of influencing regulations). In doing so, interest groups waste resources that could have otherwise been dedicated to productive activities.

Famously, Gary Becker (1983, 1985) analysed interest groups' politics in a competitive process for political influence. Competition among interest groups is argued to produce a diversity of policies and regulation swaying in several, often opposing ways, the net results of which might be an allocation of existing resources not too far from efficiency. However, when only a handful of interest groups get organised and influence the policy process, the result might be far from optimal. Olson (1965) argues that groups with more concentrated benefits and/or diffused costs are more likely to cooperate and get organised; in contrast, the ones with diffused benefits and/or concentrated costs are less likely to succeed in cooperating to influence policy and regulation. This second view is relatively more pessimistic, but can help explain why the bulk of the lobbying activity in healthcare is mainly undertaken by a small number of corporations and professional groups such as medical doctors, hospital associations and other provider-based associations rather than patient-based ones. In such a setting, one would expect high waste from unproductive rent-seeking competition and large dissipation of resources (Mueller, 2003).

Lobbying can give rise to the so-called buying of votes (so called 'pork barrel politics'), namely an exchange of votes for support, or an investment by interest groups in information provision (e.g. studies on the relative effectiveness of a drug treatment compared to the default) that can influence regulation or the policy process. Yet lobbying involves other strategies such as the direct subsidisation of legislators that pursue the same goals as those of the lobbyist (Hall and Deardorff, 2006). That said, lobbying can help humanitarian causes too. A recent example has been the political pressure of Médecins Sans Frontières in France, which successfully allowed undocumented immigrants with life-threatening conditions to remain in the country for medical treatment (Kelly et al., 2016). Similarly, lobbying by the medical professional groups has made possible the introduction of laws that require vaccination of children after three months of birth (Kelly et al., 2016). Hence, lobbying in itself does not necessarily produce an inefficient allocation of resources. On the contrary, it is institutionalised in many countries, such as the United States, where it is embedded in the first amendment of the Constitution (Spithoven, 2011). Indeed, some studies document the influence of drug companies in deals and agreements at the time of the Affordable Care Act (ACA) negotiations in the USA (McDonough, 2012).

The rent-seeking literature, which refers more to the public choice approach to institutional design (Tullock, 1967; Krueger, 1974), develops this idea that multiple groups competing through lobbying for the concession of a single monopolistic advantage, will thus waste resources, as only one, the winner of the policy contest, will obtain the desired policy. Investment in rent-seeking by interest groups is successful when they manage to attract government subsidies such as the contracts to build new hospitals, or regulations (e.g. licences or accreditation) that put certain companies and stakeholders at an advantage by demanding a legal requirement to operate in the market, thus creating barriers to entry. Such limits to competition are likely to result in higher prices and a transfer of rents to rent-seeking parties, ultimately reducing social welfare. That is, stakeholders earn an extra rent without adding any value to the patient citizen (PC), when such resources could have been used for productive activities.

When such attempts lead to a strong influence of interest groups in setting regulations, we refer to them as 'regulatory capture'. Examples of this include the approval of drugs before a full assessment of their safety and value to society is established. Other examples include examples where clientelist politics explain how minority interest groups (e.g. local elites in a small region distributing a product that does not improve people's health), manage to steer recourses towards their region in exchange for political support or political favours. The mechanisms that interest groups employ are heterogeneous too, and often include so-called revolving doors, namely offering jobs and positions in company boards to representatives and regulators that favour specific interest groups. More generally, where investing in 'favourable health regulation' is less costly than developing more efficient health services, one would expect the proliferation of activities of little value, and more generally a suboptimal use of resources in the health system. These activities deviate from corruption and bribes (even though they generate some waste) as they are intended to sway public choices but might not be necessarily inefficient. However, what they have in common is that the PC suffers a welfare loss because of such activities (Olson, 1982).

As in many other phenomena examined in this book, there is a demand and supply of rents. Bureaucrats and political incumbents might supply such rents in the form of regulations, and hence initiate the process, or interest groups might do so by offering resources in exchange. However, the consequences of rent-seeking are not trivial in a society where agents have varying power and resources, especially tax payers in the development of inequalities (Stiglitz, 2012). The rest of this chapter attempts to describe and characterise different forms of mechanisms that interest groups draw upon to exert an influence in shaping healthcare policymaking, regulation and spending.

REGULATORY CAPTURE

Regulatory capture refers to an intrinsic problem in the regulation of any kind of industry, almost without exception. Capture takes place when regulatory decisions are directed away from public interest, and instead, the regulated manages to get the regulator to cater to its interests. For example, if only one large monopolist (e.g. a major drug producer) was organised to exert pressure on a matter such as excluding a specific new treatment for coverage, its market influence might give rise to regulatory capture (Stigler, 1971; Posner, 1974; Peltzman, 1976).

Regulatory capture refers to activities that regularly attempt to sway priorities away from collective interests and to benefit particular interest groups. Such activities typically allow particular groups to extract rents (Carpenter and Moss, 2013). Officials, whether elected or not, can be influenced to change policy priorities, and more generally, their agenda by business groups and lobbyists.

However, the way capture takes place is very specific to the country's health system regulation, and it can involve rewards to research projects and conference organisations in attempts to manipulate published information, as well as more traditional problems associated with conflicts of interest. As a result, resources are misallocated away from efficiency, and encourage rent-seeking. As Angus Deaton puts it in referring to the health sector: 'It's an exquisitely designed rent-seeking mechanism, where you can seek large rents without most people understanding what you've done.'[1] The OECD (2018, p. 3) states that capture 'erodes the democratic principles of fair decision-making based on openness, dialogue, consensus and public interest'. It is especially problematic in the health sector as it limits the trust in the health system, and potentially threatens a country's health.

A common explanation of why the health system is more prone to regulatory capture and rent-seeking is that healthcare is a technically complex matter for the average PC. That is, both the regulators and regulated often do not exhibit a balanced share of power and information, especially in terms of interests, expectations and knowledge (Kwak, 2013). The way rent-seeking and regulatory capture unfolds is often unique to the dynamics of each industry, and, as we argue throughout the chapter, capture in healthcare is particularly pervasive due to the information asymmetries that provide advantages to certain providers that are effective at organising themselves to influence government decision-making (to disclose only the relevant information that benefits them), insurers and even PCs themselves (to take advantage of their health insurance contract). This explains, to a certain extent, the unique type of inefficiencies in the functioning of healthcare markets: the reasons favouring rent-seeking are also those reasons that explain why the government should

---

[1] https://promarket.org/angus-deaton-discussed-driver-inequality-america-easier-rent-seekers-affect-policy-much-europe/.

substitute the market mechanism in allocating resources in the healthcare sector.

Capture tends to take place under the so-called dilemma of collective action (Olson, 1965), namely, the more diffused the benefits within a group of individuals with a common interest, the lower the ability to organise as an interest group to promote that interest. For instance, it is not uncommon in the health sector that governmental agencies derive income from the regulated, and those who consume their services. Public agencies lack information on the direct performance indicators and hence, the regulated might hide away potential interests by the bureaucracy to inflate costs, creating a lower level of non-market output than would be efficient. This might result from the fact that bureaucrats may be budget-maximiser organisations, and that it is very difficult to obtain the relevant information on both quantities, and especially on quality of healthcare (Le Grand, 1991).

Different Faces of Regulatory Capture

Regulatory capture is hard to describe because capture adopts different forms, including 'identification with the industry, sympathy with the particular problems that regulated firms confront in meeting standards, and absence of toughness' (Makkai and Braithwaite, 1992). Interaction between regulated and the regulators might divert their preferences over time and make them prone to lobbying pressures, setting aside the wider public interest. If that happens, then the regulation corresponds more with the interests of the regulated than the wider public, which is what we define as government capture.

When one thinks in terms of regulatory capture, the first thing one can imagine is a lobbyist trying to convince the government to change the way they approach certain health-related needs, the criteria they use to regulate (e.g. cost per Quality-Adjusted Life Year, or QALY), or even the instruments they use (cost-effectiveness analysis being an example). PCs are often ignorant of the mechanisms of regulatory capture, or capture itself. As a result, the regulator does not cater to them, and instead caters to the regulated. The regulator prefers to 'err on the side of the regulated', as any mistake that entails a cost to the industry gives rise to exposure, whilst errors benefiting the industry typically are not exposed (Leaver, 2009).

Finally, another way capture makes inroads is when there are large revolving doors between regulators and professionals. Individuals who used to work for the National Health Service (NHS) become employed by pharmaceutical companies, often to carry out work in the same area of expertise they were working in as regulators. Such practices are, of course, legal and probably could be argued to be ethically acceptable, but one must recognise that they can challenge the working of a health system if they become general practice.

Information Dependence

Healthcare regulators (health insurers) depend on the information of the regulated (hospital providers) for a number of decisions, including in setting an efficient reimbursement system. That is, regulators ideally need to observe the quality of care to design a system that promotes the 'right type' of competition (Chalkley and Malcomson, 1998). This gives rise to the need to cater to providers in order for them to disclose information to be used in the regulatory process. Given the PCs' ignorance, or even limited learning potential on how the healthcare delivery works, it is not infrequent for the regulators to set regulations that do not cater for social welfare, but to the potential performance of the regulated. However, given the role of private information in the hands of the regulated agent, information disclosure becomes a source of power. Hence, regulated hospitals have little interest in disclosing information that can be used to expose them.

Bertoli and Grembi (2017) study the incidence of physicians among regional politicians to explain the variation in the use of diagnostic-related groups (DRGs) with low-technology intensity. More generally, connections with healthcare decision makers bring profits to vested interests and, in contrast, users of the health system face collective action in organising themselves to defend their own interests. However, it is a complex matter to distinguish between due and undue connections, and strategies to influence decision-making can become more sophisticated over time, such as producing information and policy research which might well not be at the service of public interests, but help specific organisations pursue their private goals. Capture takes place in shaping what is included in certain regulations, their implementation, and it can also refer to endorsement. The ultimate result is the production of a rent that could alternatively be created by market barriers to entry, such as product differentiation. However, it moves rents from society, that could otherwise be directed towards innovation, into the hands of specific interest groups.

Revolving Doors and Career Incentives

Scholars have discussed about the dangers of revolving doors as regulators can become excessively receptive to the demands of the regulated and, hence, create a source of bias (Dal Bó, 2006). However, regulatory capture of regulators is that it is difficult to measure empirically (Dal Bó, 2006; Kwak, 2013). It can be studied through campaign contributions, lobbying and employment opportunities. Interestingly, lobbying can work in two ways: first, through incentives; second, through disincentives such as trials, reputational damage or threatening to offshore jobs. Regulatory capture is not limited to regulators or supervisors specific to an industry, however, as it can also more generally involve politicians.

The difference between competition for rents and the role of a large monopolist capturing regulation is that when capture takes place, unlike rent-seeking, favours are systematically assigned to the same parties (lobbies), which can often result in the waste of resources.

As mentioned earlier, it is not infrequent in the United Kingdom to see individuals that have worked for the NHS or the National Institute for Health and Care Excellence (NICE) for some years ending up working for the pharmaceutical industry, private consultancies or the insurance sector, which is a form of revolving door albeit not an illegitimate career development. However, as we argue below, it provides perverse incentives to the functioning of healthcare markets that depend so critically on regulations. If personal contacts and private information play a role, it is inevitable that revolving doors tend to benefit the regulated industries.

The potential for 'future employment in exchange for favours' whilst acting as the regulated should be audited and shamed throughout an individual's career. Inevitably, regulators have unique knowledge of the healthcare market that the regulated might well be willing to pay for, as experience and specific organisational knowledge on loopholes in the regulation of certain healthcare industries can prove particularly profitable for the regulated.

Publication of Medical Research

One of the ways the industry can capture the regulators is by controlling certain journals, or even by having close connections to editors of certain journals in order to publish industry-friendly results which the industry can, in turn, use to lobby regulators by claiming that certain regulations are evidence-based, when alternative ones have not been adequately tested. The capture of only a few editors is enough to spread to the entire profession (Zingales, 2017). Similarly, the more specialised and disconnected from the mainstream a discipline becomes, the less costly it is for the industry to influence academic research. Researchers who are funded by the industry and carry out frequent consultancy work for it are more likely to be subject to industry pressures, as they have more to lose.

Data Access and Employment

Access to proprietary data can act to the advantage of certain agents in a competitive market. In contrast, when data is accessible by all parties, then capture through its restrictive use becomes less common, as the capacity of regulators and independent researchers to react to industry-funded research is made easier. Medicines agencies in the Western world, which authorise the entry of new medicines in their respective therapeutic markets, are mostly financed by the fees coming from new medicines applications. Hence, the industry is indirectly the main source of employment in such agencies, and a reduction in applications would result in a cutback of the staff employed by such agencies. This is an endemic problem, as bureaucrats' expectations and goals can naturally align with the interests of the industry (Niskanen, 1971). Evidence of regulatory capture is emerging in the pharmaceutical sector in the USA, and specifically the use of accelerated approval of new treatments by the Food and Drug Administration (FDA) since 1992, which is conceived of as an extraordinary application to speed up the market entry of drugs and biologics 'expected to provide a meaningful advantage over available therapies' (Naci et al., 2017). However, this procedure has become commonly used and leaves the FDA making decisions on the approval of new medicines often without sufficient data, frequently surrogate measures rather than clinical trials.

Another important example includes the role of pharmaceutical benefit managers, organisations that in the USA are set up to undertake a monopsony purchasing role. However, their contracts include the so-called gag clauses that prohibit pharmacists from telling customers that they could save money by paying cash for prescription drugs rather than using their health insurance, and the difference often goes to the benefit managers. Some US states have reacted to the problem such as the North Dakota law that states a pharmacy benefit manager or insurer may not charge a co-payment that exceeds the actual cost of a medication.

The Role of the Media

The media can play a key role in putting pressure on social stakeholders, such as patient organisations, to influence the government to change the regulation of medicines that have been delisted from the public medicines catalogue, or technologies that are not cost-effective to implement. Journalists often lack adequate skills on economics, let alone healthcare economics to understand what the effects are of not funding certain drugs (more funds for other, more necessary treatments). Given that the influence of interest groups cannot be contested in a competitive way without a transparent reporting of the private gains of specific interest groups, the role of the media in reporting on such matters can affect the extent of rent-seeking and its overall effects on the health system. If media groups are themselves influenced, or are dependent for funding, from the same interest groups that obtain private rents from government actions and regulations, then it is unlikely that the PC will be aware of the political choices that are not in their best interest.

Corporate Threats

Governments, especially weaker ones, are afraid of being regarded as 'anti-business', and they prefer to err on the side of the interests of large corporations. An example is the so-called private finance initiative (PFI), a public procurement mechanism where private firms are contracted to complete and manage public infrastructural projects, such as new hospitals in a partnership, which has been extensively used in the UK, Australia and Spain. The public sector sets the specifications and then, once completed, has to pay back within a period normally of twenty to forty years. Given that the costs come later, the current government would not be politically penalised if the private use of such infrastructures turned out not to be efficient (Ball et al., 2001). Another advantage is that the costs of setting up new infrastructures do not add to public debt. Hence, blurs the PC capacity to build wicksellian connections.

Although presented as a means for increasing accountability and efficiency, PFIs have increased the NHS debt and have been labelled by the UK National Audit Office as being more expensive (House of Commons, 2011), while mostly not realising the benefits hoped for (National Audit Office, 2018). Although introduced by the

Conservative government, PFIs became widespread and became the main method of building new hospitals in the UK in labour governments. During the financial crises, the NHS trusts had to fund the PFI itself by lending money to private organisations. In contrast, in Scotland, the model was carried out using a non-profit-distributing vehicle which would cap private sector returns.

LOBBYING AND RENT-SEEKING IN HEALTHCARE

There is growing empirical evidence of the importance of lobbying and rent-seeking in healthcare. Kushel and Bindman (2004) provide an early review on the topic. For example, Carpenter et al. (1998) analyse lobbying networks in US healthcare and find support on 'network effects', in other words lobbyists' access is dependent on the access of other related lobbyists. Cooper et al. (2017) show that US hospitals that were recipients of Section 508 policy, allowing them to waive Medicare reimbursements, did form a hospital coalition, spending millions of dollars in lobbying Congress for the programme's extension. This type of lobbying activity materialised in a 22 per cent increase in campaign contributions for those Congressmen elected in districts with a '508 policy' hospital recipient. The percentage rose to 65 per cent when looking at individual contributions of those working in the healthcare sector.

In the contexts of the negotiation of the ACA, Spithoven (2016) found evidence of effective collective lobbying involvement, which supported the reform after in exchange of to influencing its design. Landers and Sehgal (2004) provided an early account of total lobbying spending in healthcare of $237 million in 2000, 15 per cent of total federal lobbying, exceeding lobbying spending in any other sectors. Perhaps not surprisingly, they also found that within the healthcare sector, pharmaceutical and health product companies were those spending the most ($96 million). These companies were then followed by physicians and other health professionals ($46 million), and disease advocacy and public health organisation groups, which spent about $12 million. They also found a sharp increase in lobbying from depending on the specific health-related groups. Landers and Sehgal (2000) explored the role of Senate and House legislative assistants and their meetings with, respectively, ten and four physicians per month. Common topics discussed in such meetings were Medicare reimbursement, managed care reform and funding for medical research. Perhaps surprisingly, issues such as access to care for the uninsured, tobacco control, abortion rights and violence prevention were rarely discussed.

Similarly, in the context of ACA approval, the initially planned Medicaid drug prices were revisited in exchange for support to the reform and the provision of extension of discounts for certain Medicare recipients, and proposals to allow drug reimportation did not pass Senate approval (Spithoven, 2016). Other proposals to speed up the introduction of generic drugs, however, did manage to get the approval of Congress (Jaffe, 2015).

Overall, this evidence suggests that lobbying does indeed manage to exert some influence and change policy, as well as regulation. However, consistently with Olson (1965), the effects of lobbying seem to be asymmetric, as smaller groups and those with less concentrated benefits are at a disadvantage in influencing legislators given that they are less likely to be effectively organised and, if they are, they might be able to bear the costs of lobbying activities.

SUMMARY

The health sector is particularly prone to the influence of interest groups, which attempt to lobby legislators, compete for favours, and sometimes manage to capture the government with the promotion of rent-producing regulations in the form of monopolistic profits and swaying resources away from the PC's best interest. Also, if the deadweight loss from the regulation-based monopoly power created under capture is small, certainly the transfer of large amounts of surplus from patients to healthcare companies and providers, poses non-negligible moral and ethical questions about equity and fairness. Normative analysis, requiring the comparison of utilities of agents, might then be required for judging such activities.

Not all lobbying gives rise to government failure. On the contrary, health insurance extensions and the introduction of important health policies have been the direct consequence of lobbying activities. However, the health sector provides a significant scope for profit-making given the growing demand of healthcare motivated by the extension of life expectancy and the increasing expectation of the quality of life on the part of citizens and voters.

Interest group activities, in the form of lobbying or other types of pressure, are common, important and salient in healthcare policy-making. In this chapter we gave several examples of them. With the progressive involvement of the government in health, we should expect interest groups in healthcare to be more and more active in shaping policy and public decision-making. As most of healthcare is provided in the form of individual curative medicine, it can be excluded from public funding and provided and financed by the market. This opens up the prospects for commercial healthcare activities being built around the public intervention in healthcare. Interests groups can benefit from small changes in regulation and policy. Hence, it is not surprising that private sector interests target the health sector with the expectation of profiting out of it. The example of the negotiations of the ACA suggests that lobbying succeeded in pursuing the interests of the pharmaceutical industry, the medical and nursing professions, as well as insurance organisations (Spithoven, 2016). However, the welfare effects for the median PC are not always straightforward to identify, and there is scope for institutional design to limit the negative consequences of lobbying and rent-seeking by increasing transparency alongside encouraging competition between public and private actors.

In this chapter we stressed how not all lobbying wastes resources. There are, however, important points to make. The first is stemming from regulatory capture. As capture creates large rents in the form of transfers, there will be most pressing demands in terms of fairness, equity and access in healthcare in the future on the part of the PC. Second, while capture might be economically inefficient, deadweight losses might not be large. However, rent-seeking theory tells us that there is potential for vast waste of resources in healthcare as all the activities to obtain these transfers – forms of 'all-in' auctions – will be conducted at progressively higher opportunity costs, with the risk of dissipating those rents themselves.

10 Political Sustainability of Health Innovation

THE POLITICAL VALUE OF INNOVATION

As health has been made both more effective and expensive by medical advances, it has raised political concerns in terms of how to sustain such improvements and, at the same time, guarantee access to them by the patient citizen (PC). Concerns about the sustainability of increasing health expenditures through time are at a trade-off with the expansions in the quality and quantity of life, which, especially in wealthy societies, are much more valued than expansions in consumption and income. In this chapter, we look at how three standard models (electoral models, power dominance and lobbying) have been theoretically introduced and empirically tested in the field of health innovation. We argue that innovations in health are subject to increasing political scrutiny by the PC, and this can give rise to dramatic changes in the political incentives of voters, interest groups and branches of government.

When considering the tremendous evolution that healthcare systems, goods and services have undergone in the last few decades, it is difficult not to think about medical innovation. Innovation in health is naturally connected to health R&D which, deeply shapes healthcare provision and interacts with health insurance. The interplay among these dimensions – the so-called quadrilemma – is central in defining the types, evolution and challenges for health systems around the world (Weisbrod, 1991; Costa-Font et al., 2012).[1]

---

[1] While there are many advances in lifestyle and consumption habits that have a substantial effect on people's health, most of the innovation we will refer to in this chapter is *curative medicine* embodied in goods and services typically supplied by healthcare providers, so that the advance makes healthcare more effective in

From a broad perspective, we can state that medical progress affects medical expenditures through three main channels. It influences (i) healthcare prices, (ii) individual patients' utilisation (individual intensive margin) and throughout the life cycle (individual extensive margin) and (iii) diffusion (patient extensive margin) of healthcare usage among a larger share of potential patients.

(i) Examples of *price/cost* effects can stem from increased costs of development and patenting from regulatory systems of approvals and standards of quality around medical innovation; or by drawing from progressively higher opportunity costs resources to drive innovation. This is in part due to regulation or bottlenecks in the input factors of research. Moreover, as new ideas are just more difficult to find (Bloom et al., 2017), innovation will be more expensive to produce, and the amounts and costs of resources to apply in R&D to sustain the rate of innovation will rise as well.

(ii) Innovation might cause *increasing utilisation* of healthcare on the part of patients if new drugs and therapies complement, more than substitute, the existing ones, for example to relieve the side effects of main therapies (intensive margin). This is also related to the overall increase in usage for an individual as ageing and chronicity, for example, imply a larger use of healthcare goods and services throughout the life cycle (extensive margin).

(iii) An example of an *extensive margin* is one of increasing diffusion of therapies transforming people affected by disease into treatable 'patients'. Another strategy lies in finding new applications of drugs or health devices to other diseases and health conditions that were not originally intended to be addressed by new drugs or other type of medical innovation.[2]

improving the quality and quantity of life (see Solow, 1962; Lichtenberg and Virabhak, 2002 for an application to the healthcare sector).

[2] Finally, while there is often focus on drug and devices innovation, it is worth noting that an extensive definition would also include *organisational innovation* as a method, for example, to organise the supply and utilisation of existing health goods and services in a new and more efficient way, without reducing the health impact of the existing healthcare. These types of innovation are usually focused on reducing costs more than increasing benefits, and will ultimately result in declining usage and thus expenditures without affecting the quality of and impact on health outcomes.

The final effect of technology on healthcare expenditures will thus depend on how innovation affects the cost, use and diffusion of healthcare. The relative roles of these channels in contributing to the growth of healthcare expenditures can be gauged by looking at how biomedical R&D is pushed towards certain objectives, for example through the effect of tax cuts or direct subsidisation, as well as using tax cuts for private R&D. The costs of innovation will depend also on the likelihood that public or private insurers will cover the innovation once it is available in the market, by expected demographic shifts in the population (Acemoglu and Linn, 2004), or by the disease incidence dynamics. Also, by changes in the rules governing the actors of the overall existing health system, by income growth or on the specific patenting system in use, just to give some examples.

While it is often challenging to disentangle the relative contributions just discussed, the overall effect of innovation seems to indicate a substantial positive impact on health expenditures. Research finds that health innovation is the predominant driver of health spending when also considering other variables such as income or insurance coverage (Newhouse, 1992; Okunade and Murthy, 2002; Chernew and Newhouse, 2012; Atella and Kopinska, 2018). For example, also when innovation decreases per-unit costs, the expansion in the new treatment's diffusion might be enough to increase overall expenditures. This trend, which is sharp in the USA, has been substantial also across other developed countries (Barros, 1998; Dybczak and Przywara, 2010; see also Figure 10.1).

The 'large' growth rate – meaning larger than that of the GDP – resulted in economies progressively spending an increasing portion of their total product on the consumption of healthcare. This is the progression of healthcare *excess spending,* as proposed in Squires (2014), and in Chen and Goldman (2016) (see Figure 10.2). One view is that health technology has made healthcare to take up a greater share of our budgets, but this has happened, on average, with a large and positive impact on patients' welfare (Cutler and McClellan, 2001;

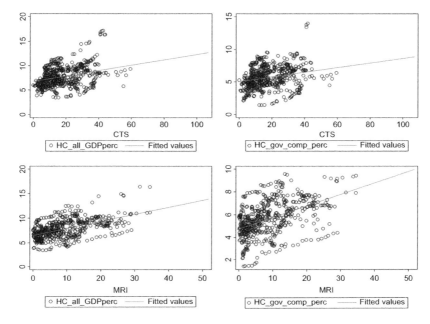

FIGURE 10.1 Correlations between health spending (total and public) and health technology diffusion: Computed Tomography Scan (CTS, top panels), and Magnetic Resonance Imaging (MRI, bottom panels)

Murphy and Topel, 2003a, 2006; Cutler, 2007). Certainly, today we live longer (quantity) and healthier (quality) lives than our grandparents and ancestors did not more than a century ago. A great part of these achievements is predicated on the availability of what is today a wide spectrum of treatments unthinkable only a few decades ago: drugs, devices, procedures and modalities of care, which have made our relationship with illness and health risks way easier to deal with than in the relatively recent past.

It has also been suggested that medical innovation showing very marginal effects on people's health does represent the best option to allocate spending with the highest welfare impact. To explain why this is the case, this effect has been driven by income growth and the shift in preferences for health, with the result of putting a very high value – in terms of marginal contribution to one's utility – on the

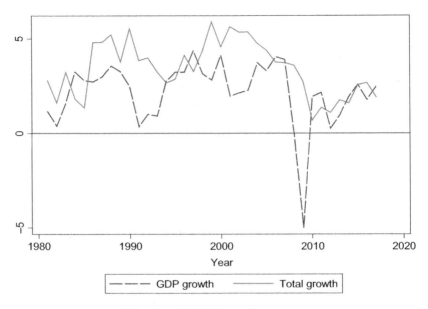

FIGURE 10.2 'Excess' total health spending
Note: OECD health data from 2019 comparing health and GDP growth
rates from 1980 to 2017.

quality and quantity of life with respect to increasing consumption. If
so, a larger share of health spending on GDP should just give rise to a
welfare gain from health innovation without creating concerns for a
country's public and private finances. Perhaps, in fact, larger welfare
gains are on the horizon, and evidence of the suboptimal levels of
today's health spending is available. For example, Hall and Jones
(2007) suggest that the optimal spending in healthcare in the USA
might well converge towards 30 per cent of the GDP in the near
future, and with large welfare gains.

There seems to be, however, some evidence that not all innovation provides real improvement to patients and can waste resources,
with consequential mistreatment and overtreatment. Similarly, there
are several instances where innovation has produced very limited
benefits, and this to the point of questioning its worthiness. The
existence of substantial pockets of waste and mismanagement (as

reported in Chapter 8) have raised the question about what best measures would need to be taken to avoid superfluous costs from administering unnecessary treatment (Lyu et al., 2017).

A common form of evidence comes from geographical variations in healthcare spending per patient which is rarely associated with comparable health outcomes. An early analysis is Eddy (1984), while for a more recent review of the literature on the topic, see Skinner (2011). To be clear, some variation must be allowed, and not necessarily respond to the existence of medical waste. Variations in practice might just reflect searching for continuous improvements and maintaining comparative advantages in expertise and quality of healthcare across providers. Indeed, the application of many innovations that might respond well in clinical trials might need to be *fine-tuned* when used in the field within the supply of actual treatments, at a vast scale, and by highly heterogeneous organisations of providers. This can be at the source of uncertainty and waste, but is likely to be reduced through time as best practices of delivery administration are perfected and diffused, while new ones are introduced selectively at the beginning. Overall, the interplay of these competitive and learning mechanisms should not be blamed for producing unnecessary care, but quite the opposite. However, this evidence might also reveal the existence of systematic allocative inefficiency of medical resources. Chandra and Staiger (2017) study the practice of reperfusion as a consequence of myocardial infarction and find evidence both of comparative advantage in supplying healthcare, but also of substantial waste from allocative inefficiency in the USA.

A critical factor behind this inefficiency is the ability to optimally manage an ever-evolving set of healthcare treatments depending on technology types and management procedures that should address correctly the target population of patients (Chandra and Skinner, 2012). The expensive nature of healthcare and its impact on health and resource waste potential crucially depend on its embodied technology. Some technology makes this matching easy, other technology is more likely to produce mismatching, ultimately producing the misuse of health treatments and the consequent waste of healthcare resources.

POLITICAL DRIVERS OF HEALTH TECHNOLOGY

One consequence of the availability and spread of life-saving and financially expensive treatments is the standardisation of provision of healthcare. It has been noted that the initial introduction of expensive and life-saving innovations has the effect of exacerbating the *health-gradient inequality*, which is the strong empirical regularity of a positive correlation between income and life expectancy or other measures of health outcomes (Deaton, 2002). This effect can plausibly engender a political demand from the median voter to reduce such imbalance. These programmes usually seek to improve access to medical care by providing insurance or through the direct supply of healthcare through a national system. Indeed, there is some evidence that public healthcare reduces differentials in life expectancy between high- and low-income groups.

However, as described in Chapter 6, the use of median voter equilibria is not so intuitive; as inequality might, in fact, give rise to an *ends against the middle equilibrium* where both the poor and the wealthy vote against public provision.[3] In short, medical innovation has been crucial both in determining health spending, as well as many of the characteristics of health systems, and in deciding the respective roles (interactions/interdependencies) of the public and private sectors which, in turn, depend on political factors on both the side of the voters and that of the interest groups. Topel (2017) argues that policy changes influence the *downstream* perspectives of innovating companies in terms of expected market demand and diffusion of treatments.

An important political driver of medical innovation is through its direct subsidisation. Direct subsidisation occurs also, and through

---

[3] The specific equilibrium emerging will depend on the specific assumptions modelling the electoral politics.

public R&D spending. One typical example is the US National Institutes of Health (NIH), whose budget exceeds $30 billion dollars in total funding per year. Publicly subsidised R&D sustains innovation from public institutions, and it is also found to be complementary to private R&D spending in the pharmaceutical industry. Toole (2007) provides evidence that public medical R&D stimulates and complements private medical R&D, though with heterogeneous size and time effects. This is also demonstrated to be true for payment systems and regulation, with both theoretical and empirical analysis (Baumgartner, 1991; Caudill et al., 1995; Baker, 2001), and, of course, for patenting law, which heavily influences incentives in innovation as well by granting monopoly rights for a predetermined amount of time.

Lewis Thomas Early View

An early approach linking health technology to the social and political factors that might affect it, is from Lewis Thomas (1975, 1977, 1988).

Thomas argues that the type of technology resulting from medical R&D depends on the balance between basic and applied research. There are two types of technology: half-way technology and high technology.[4] The first type is the result of applied research; it tends to produce results in the shorter term and is dedicated to the suppression of symptoms more than cure of the underlying causes of the disease, which have not yet been well understood. In contrast, high technology originates instead from the production of basic scientific knowledge, which sheds light on the underlying causes of the disease and supplies very effective technology at relatively low costs. However, basic research has its own costs, because it will tend to produce results in the long term, and with more uncertain outcomes.

---

[4] In the same article, Lewis Thomas talks also about a baseline type called *non-technology*, which is the case where treatments are basically ineffective palliative cures, but adopted anyway in the absence of better options.

Thus, in the presence of this trade-off, what will be observed is a combination of research types. A more applied than basic combination will produce more halfway than high technology and vice versa. While Thomas does not develop his thinking into a model of political economy, in his 1977 and 1988 articles, he discusses the public incentives to have ready-to-use/halfway technology. For example, he writes that, 'Medicine is expected to do something for each of these illnesses, to do whatever can be done in the light of today's knowledge. Because of this obligation, "halfway" technologies have evolved, representing the best available treatment ... but at a very high cost and with considerable waste resulting from overuse' (Thomas, 1988, p. 303).

In other terms, social and political demands for ready-to-use solutions, perhaps depending on the biased view of the public's little faith in long-term biological research outcomes, imply that healthcare is using readily available knowledge to respond to the most pressing health problems of the day. The political demand for ready-to-apply results from medical research tilts the balance towards more applied research, with the observed results in terms of health technology.[5] A similar view has come from different perspectives of imperatives, of quasi-lexicographic preferences.

---

[5] Another way to capture Thomas's view is saying that, from this perspective, existing knowledge is fixed in supply and it is not a pure public good, but a common resource. Basic research expands the pool of ideas for potential innovation, while applied research draws from it, but with decreasing marginal chances for successful innovation. Thus, finding successful applications becomes progressively harder for applied research. Access is free, but the number of inventions that can be drawn depends on the number of useful combinations that can be drawn. The public demand for improved health encourages research projects producing improvements in the short run. Most of the applied research draws from a fixed body of existing knowledge to produce innovations. As knowledge is fixed, there is a sort of *tragedy of the commons* because its exploitation on the part of applied researchers makes it gradually more difficult to find new ideas to produce substantial innovation and welfare. There is a clear trade-off between focusing more on short-run research, which is more likely to produce halfway technology, and long-run results, which have the potential to produce high technology, but whose results are more uncertain and likely to be expected over the longer term.

Electoral Models

More recently, electoral models have been extended to include health technology. Bethencourt and Galasso (2008) propose a median voter equilibrium, showing the *complementarity between pension and public healthcare programmes*. They assume the health gradient, in other words that longevity and income are positively correlated in the population. Public healthcare programmes have the effect of increasing voters' longevity, more strongly that of low-income voters than high-income ones, which has the effect of mitigating the health gradient itself. The overall result is that the increase in pensions payments will be more directed towards low-income voters. In other terms, improved longevity will make social security relatively more attractive for low-income voters, which will give political support to social security expansions. Finally, this complementarity is strengthened by medical innovation. Innovative health technology increases the longevity gains from public healthcare spending, and increased longevity furtherly promotes the rise of pensions' expenditures following the same mechanism illustrated above.

Alternatively, Moreno-Ternero and Roemer (2010) propose an electoral model explaining the interaction between two parties, one on the left and the other on the right, which need to decide if and how to cover cost-increasing medical innovation. The paper shows that, in the political equilibrium proposed, both parties will vote to cover the latest and most expensive innovation. However, the left-wing party, representing low-income voters, will decide to do so through public spending, while the right-wing party will support private spending. The political compromise will finance cost-increasing innovation with a mix of public and private healthcare spending, which explains the rise in overall health expenditures because of medical innovation.

Finally, Batinti and Congleton (2018) consider medical technology as endogenous, and as dependent on political support for medical R&D. They then explore the interaction between medical R&D subsidisation and public health insurance, in other words the interplay between the political demands for better care on the one hand, and access to care on the other. When R&D produces innovation leading to growth in health expenditures, the political demand for public insurance is found to increase. The consequences of these interactions depend on the respective median voters' responses when voting on the two dimensions of public R&D and public health insurance. One possibility is that expenditure-increasing R&D is supported by voters if they expect resulting medical treatments to be publicly subsidised.

Congressional Dominance

There is also research focusing on the power that political institutions exert in incentivising funding of specific agencies to increase or consolidate their political power. This also includes funding for medical innovation. Some important empirical work explores the political economy of the NIH. NIH funding has steadily grown during the last decade, and today its budget exceed $30 billion per year. This funding is mainly attributed to competitive grants for extramural research by the different institutes, and promotes the discovery and development of new medical treatments and technologies, while stimulating private medical R&D. However, its dynamics are driven by the presence of congressional and presidential dominance.

According to models of the industrial organisation of legislature, such as the one proposed in Weingast and Marshall (1988), Congress organises committees to facilitate decision-making and redistributes power among politicians according to the committee they are assigned to. As Congress is organised in several committees, the ones that have a major influence on the NIH budget are the House and Senate appropriations committees. Politicians in key committees thus 'control' or 'dominate' the bureaucratic bodies or agencies under their jurisdiction, and control of their funding is implied as well. Research explores the congressional dominance hypothesis looking at the role of 'power' committees in Congress in directing the NIH funding towards states/districts that are of interest for electoral reasons (Hegde and Mowery, 2008; Hegde, 2009; Sampat, 2012).

Hegde (2009) looks at the distribution of NIH grants by performer according to the location in a certain congressional district. Hegde finds that performers in congressional districts represented by both a House or Senate member of the Appropriation Committees and a member of the Labor and Health relative subcommittees receive, on average, 6–10 per cent more funding while controlling for a series of other confounding factors and performers' fixed effects. Godefroy (2011) follows a similar line of empirical inquiry and studies the composition of specific groups in Congress, in other words committees, subcommittees and parties, and explores their power in directing NIH funds towards clinical research that deals with diseases that constitute an important burden (measured as the impact on life years lost) on their districts. It is found that the House Subcommittee on Labor, Health and Human Services has an important impact on funding towards clinical research (research involving humans in clinical trials) across diseases, while no effect is found when looking at basic research.

Presidential Dominance

Even though the congressional dominance view is suggestive, it has nonetheless been put under scrutiny and criticism (Moe, 1987; Moe and Wilson, 1994). It has been proposed that the role of the executive branch, the President in particular, has oversight power, and possesses instruments of political leverage to affect agencies' decision-making as well. As the legislative branch of government affects NIH distribution granting through the committee structure, so the executive power of the president has channels to influence, if not directly, the funding of the NIH. Batinti (2016), for example, looks as well at the distribution of the NIH funding received by swing voter states during presidential elections from 1972 to 2012. The paper finds empirical support for presidential dominance, as swing voter states in presidential elections receive between 7 and 10 per cent more funds.

Lobbying for Rare Diseases

One aspect of lobbying on medical R&D is that related to rare diseases. Research has shown the effect of policymaking on rare disease R&D funding. Yin (2008) explores the effects of the tax credits for drug development targeting rare diseases established by the 1983 Orphan Drug Act (ODA). The author finds that the introduction of supply-side subsidisation increased innovative activity (measured by new clinical trials for a large group of rare diseases), and on average found that the ODA led to a 69 per cent increase in the annual flow of new clinical trials for rare diseases. Recent research also documents lobbying the NIH to obtain policies supporting rare disease research. Hegde and Sampat (2015) analyse the lobbying behaviour of pressure groups advocating for NIH funding for rare diseases. Lobbying promotes political support in the form of *soft-earmarking* on the part of Congress. Soft-earmarking is used to drive NIH funding towards the rare disease advocated, and influence is also consistent with scientific opportunity and disease burden. This indicates that lobbying does not necessarily distort funding from the most effective use, but has an informational role to promote funding towards those diseases – within the set of rare ones – that helps direct NIH funding towards the 'best' use. In other words, lobbying is found to be effective to advocate for funding when there is higher scientific opportunity (number of scientific publications related to the study of the disease) and disease burden (measured by number of deaths caused by the disease).[6]

SUMMARY

In this chapter we have shown that medical innovation is central in the development of healthcare systems, and hence for the well-being of the PC. More specifically, 'push' factors (of medical innovation) have mostly focused on the politics of NIH funding for the USA and equivalent agencies elsewhere. This has been because the NIH is the

---

[6] For evidence on disease burden as NIH driver, see also Sampat et al. (2013).

world's largest funder for biomedical R&D, and for data availability as well. In contrast, 'pull' factors might be explained by the diffusion of health insurance programmes which are based, though not exclusively, on median voter-type models. This diffusion influences jointly the rate of development of technology, the size of public healthcare programmes and health spending overall.

Finally, new perspectives from technology in healthcare, genetics, genomics, digital health and personalised care are promising future fields of study. These innovations will impact both the cost nature of new technologies but will also affect the welfare contributions from insurance as they have the potential to deeply transform the way in which healthcare is consumed throughout the life-cycle of the patient citizen.

Bibliography

Acemoglu, D. and Johnson, S. (2007). Disease and development: The effect of life expectancy on economic growth. *Journal of Political Economy*, 115(6), 925–85.

Acemoglu, D. and Linn, J. (2004). Market size in innovation: Theory and evidence from the pharmaceutical industry. *The Quarterly Journal of Economics*, 119(3), 1049–90.

Acemoglu, D. and Robinson, J. A. (2000). Why did the West extend the franchise? Democracy, inequality, and growth in historical perspective. *The Quarterly Journal of Economics*, 115(4), 1167–99.

Acemoglu, D. and Robinson, J. A. (2001). A theory of political transitions. *American Economic Review*, 91(4), 938–63.

Acemoglu, D. and Robinson, J. A. (2005). *Economic Origins of Dictatorship and Democracy*. Cambridge: Cambridge University Press.

Acemoglu, D. and Robinson, J. A. (2013). *Why Nations Fail: The Origins of Power, Prosperity, and Poverty*. New York: Broadway Business.

Acemoglu, D. and Verdier, T. (1998). Property rights, corruption and the allocation of talent: A general equilibrium approach. *Economic Journal*, 18(450), 1381–403.

Acemoglu, D., Johnson, S., Robinson, J. A. and Yared, P. (2009). Reevaluating the modernization hypothesis. *Journal of Monetary Economics*, 56(8), 1043–58.

Acemoglu, D., Naidu, S., Restrepo, P. and Robinson, J. A. (2015). Democracy, redistribution, and inequality. In A. Atkinson and F. Bourguignon (eds.), *Handbook of Income Distribution* (Vol. 2). Amsterdam: Elsevier, pp. 1885–966.

Acemoglu, D., Akcigit, U., Alp, H., Bloom, N. and Kerr, W. (2018). Innovation, reallocation, and growth. *American Economic Review*, 108(11), 3450–91.

Acemoglu, D., Naidu, S., Restrepo, P. and Robinson, J. A. (2019). Democracy does cause growth. *Journal of Political Economy*, 127(1), 47–100.

Aidt, T. S. (2003). Economic analysis of corruption: A survey. *Economic Journal*, 113, F632–52.

Alesina, A., Glaeser, E. and Sacerdote, B. (2001). Why doesn't the United States have a European welfare state? *Brookings Paper on Economic Activity* (Fall), 187–278.

Alesina, A., Stantcheva, S. and Teso, E. (2018). Intergenerational mobility and preferences for redistribution. *American Economic Review*, 108(2), 521–54.

Altman, D., Flavin, P. and Radcliff, B. (2017). Democratic institutions and subject-ive well-being. *Political Studies*, 65(3), 685–704.

Amrith, S. (2001). Democracy, globalization and health: The African dilemma. Cambridge, UK: Centre for History and Economics. www.histecon.magd.cam .ac.uk/docs/amrith_healthafrica.pdf.

Anderberg, D. (1999). Determining the mix of public and private provision of insurance by majority rule. *European Journal of Political Economy*, 15(3), 417–40.

Anderson, K. M. (2015). *Social Policy in the European Union*. London: Palgrave.

Arrow, K. J. (1963). Uncertainty and the welfare economics of medical care. *American Economic Review*, 53(5), 941–73.

Arulampalam, W., Dasgupta, S., Dhillon, A. and Dutta, B. (2009). Electoral goals and centre-state transfers: A theoretical model and empirical evidence from India. *Journal of Development Economics*, 88(1), 103–19.

Atella, V. and Kopinska, J. (2018). New technologies and costs. CEIS Research Paper No. 442, Tor Vergata University.

Azfar, O. and Gurgur, T. (2008). Does corruption affect health outcomes in the Philippines? *Economics of Governance*, 9(3), 197–244.

Baicker, K. and Skinner, J. (2010). Health care spending growth and the future of US tax rates. Prepared for the NBER's 25th Tax Policy and the Economy conference, Washington, DC, 23 September 2010.

Baicker, K., Clemens, J. and Singhal, M. (2012). The rise of the states: US fiscal decentralization in the postwar period. *Journal of Public Economics*, 96(11–12), 1079–91.

Baker, L. C. (2001). Managed care and technology adoption in health care: Evidence from magnetic resonance imaging. *Journal of Health Economics*, 20, 395–421.

Balestrino, A. (1999). The desirability of in-kind transfers in the presence of distor-tionary taxes. *Journal of Economic Surveys*, 13(4), 333–54.

Ball, R., Heafey, M. and King, D. (2001). Private finance initiative – A good deal for the public purse or a drain on future generations? *Policy & Politics*, 29(1), 95–108.

Bandiera, O., Prat, A. and Valletti, T. (2009). Active and passive waste in govern-ment spending: Evidence from a policy experiment. *American Economic Review*, 99(4), 1278–308.

Banting, K. and Costa-Font, J. (2010). Decentralization, welfare, and social citizen-ship in contemporary democracies. *Environment and Planning C: Government and Policy*, 28(3), 381–8.

Barigozzi, F. and Turati, G. (2012). Human health care and selection effects: Under-standing labour supply in the market for nursing. *Health Economics*, 21(4), 477–83.

Barlow, J., Roehrich, J. K. and Wright, S. (2010). De facto privatisation or a renewed role for the EU? Paying for Europe's healthcare infrastructure in a recession. *Journal of the Royal Society of Medicine*, 103, 51–5.

Barr, N. A. (2001). *The Welfare State as Piggy Bank: Information, Risk, Uncertainty, and the Role of the State*. Oxford: Oxford University Press.

Barros, P. P. (1998). The black box of health care expenditure growth determinants. *Health Economics*, 7, 533–44.

Baskaran, T. and Hessami, Z. (2017). Political alignment and intergovernmental transfers in parliamentary systems: Evidence from Germany. *Public Choice*, 171(1), 75–98.

Batinti, A. (2016). NIH biomedical funding: Evidence of executive dominance in swing-voter states during presidential elections. *Public Choice*, 168(3–4), 239–63.

Batinti, A. and Congleton, R. D. (2018). On the codetermination of tax-financed medical R&D and healthcare expenditures: Models and evidence. *The European Journal of Political Economy*, 54(C), 175–88.

Batinti, A., Costa-Font, J. and Hatton, T. J. (2019). Voting up? The effects of democracy and franchise extension on human stature. IZA Working Paper No. 12389.

Baumgartner, J. R. (1991). The interaction between forms of insurance contract and types of technical change in medical care. *The RAND Journal of Economics*, 22(1), 36–53.

Beaglehole, R., Bonita, R., Horton, C. et al. (2011). Priority actions for the non-communicable disease crisis. *The Lancet*, 377(9775), 1438–47.

Becker, G. S. (1983). A theory of competition among pressure groups for political influence. *The Quarterly Journal of Economics*, 98(3), 371–400.

Becker, G. S. (1985). Public policies, pressure groups, and dead weight costs. *Journal of Public Economics*, 28(3), 329–47.

Becker, G. S., Philipson, T. J. and Soares, R. R. (2005). The quantity and quality of life and the evolution of world inequality. *American Economic Review*, 95(1), 277–91.

Benatar, S. R. (2002). Ethics and tropical diseases: Some global considerations. In G. Cook and A. Zumla (eds.), *Manson's Tropical Diseases*, 21st edn. Edinburgh: Elsevier Sciences, pp. 85–93.

Benz, M. and Frey, B. S. (2008). Being independent is a great thing: Subjective evaluations of self-employment and hierarchy. *Economica*, 75(298), 362–83.

Berggren, N., Jordahl, H. and Poutvaara, P. (2010). The looks of a winner: Beauty and electoral success. *Journal of Public Economics*, 94(1–2), 8–15.

Berry, K., Allen, T., Horan, R. D., Shogren, J. F., Finnoff, D. and Daszak, P. (2018). The economic case for a pandemic fund. *EcoHealth*, 1–15.

Bertoli, P. and Grembi, V. (2017). The political economy of diagnosis-related groups. *Social Science & Medicine*, 190(C), 38–47.

Berwick, D. M. and Hackbarth, D. (2012). Eliminating waste in US healthcare. *JAMA*, 307(14), 1513–16.

Besley, T. (2004). Welfare economics and public choice. In C. K. Rowley and F. Schneider (eds.), *The Encyclopedia of Public Choice*. Boston, MA: Springer, pp. 933–7.

Besley, T. (2006). *Principled Agents?: The Political Economy of Good Government*. Oxford: Oxford University Press.

Besley, T. and Case, A. (1993). Does electoral accountability affect economic policy choices? Evidence from gubernatorial term limits. NBER Working Paper No. 4575.

Besley, T. and Case, A. (2003). Political institutions and policy choices: Evidence from the United States. *Journal of Economic Literature*, 41(1), 7–73.

Besley, T. and Gouveia, M. (1994). Alternative systems of health care provision. *Economic Policy*, 9(19), 199–258.

Besley, T. and Kudamatsu, M. (2006). Health and democracy. *American Economic Review Papers and Proceedings*, 96, 313–18.

Besley, T., Hall, J. and Preston, I. (1999). The demand for private health insurance: Do waiting lists matter? *Journal of Public Economics*, 72(2), 155–81.

Betancourt, R. and Gleason, S. (2000). The allocation of publicly-provided goods to rural households in India: On some consequences of caste, religion and democracy. *World Development*, 28(12), 2169–82.

Bethencourt, C. and Galasso, V. (2008). Political complements in the welfare state: Health care and social security. *Journal of Public Economics*, 92(3–4), 609–32.

Bhalotra, S. and Clots-Figueras, I. (2014). Health and the political agency of women. *American Economic Journal: Economic Policy*, 6(2), 164–97.

Black, D. (1948). On the rationale of group decision-making. *Journal of Political Economy*, 56(1), 23–34.

Blaydes, L. and Kayser, M. A. (2011). Counting calories: Democracy and distribution in the developing world. *International Studies Quarterly*, 55(4), 887–908.

Bloom, D. E., Cadarette, D. and Sevilla, J. P. (2018). Epidemics and economics. *Finance & Development*, 55(2), 834–41.

Bloom, N., Jones, C. I., Van Reenen, J. and Webb, M. (2017). Are ideas getting harder to find? NBER Working Paper No. 23782.

Blouin, C., Chopra, M. and van der Hoeven, R. (2009). Trade and social determinants of health. *The Lancet*, 373(9662), 502–7.

Boix, C., Miller, M. and Rosato, S. (2013). A complete data set of political regimes, 1800–2007. *Comparative Political Studies*, 46(12), 1523–54.

Bollyky, T. J., Templin, T., Cohen, M., Schoder, D., Dieleman, J. L. and Wigley, S. (2019). The relationships between democratic experience, adult health, and cause-specific mortality in 170 countries between 1980 and 2016: An observational analysis. *The Lancet*, 393(10181), 1628–40.

Borck, R. (2007). Voting, inequality and redistribution. *Journal of Economic Surveys*, 21(1), 90–109.

Borck, R. (2018). Political participation and the welfare state. CESifo Working Paper No. 7128. CESifo Group Munich.

Bordignon, M. and Turati, G. (2009). Bailing out expectations and public health expenditure. *Journal of Health Economics*, 28(2), 305–21.

Bordignon, M., Colombo, L. and Galmarini, U. (2008). Fiscal federalism and lobbying. *Journal of Public Economics*, 92(12), 2288–301.

Bowen, H. R. (1943). The interpretation of voting in the allocation of economic resources. *Quarterly Journal of Economics*, 58, 27–48.

Brennan, G. and Buchanan, J. (1980). *Power to Tax: Analytical Foundations of a Fiscal Constitution*. Cambridge: Cambridge University Press.

Brennan, G. and Buchanan, J. M. (1985). *The Reason of Rules: Constitutional Political Economy*. Cambridge: Cambridge University Press.

Breton, A. (1996). *Competitive Governments: An Economic Theory of Politics and Public Finance*. New York: Cambridge University Press.

Breton, A. and Fraschini, A. (2003). Vertical competition in unitary states: The case of Italy. *Public Choice*, 114, 57–77.

Breton, A. and Scott, A. (1978). *Economic Constitution of Federal States*. Toronto: University of Toronto Press.

Breyer, F. (1995). The political economy of rationing in social health insurance. *Journal of Population Economics*, 8(2), 137–48.

Brownlee, S., Chalkidou, K., Doust, J. et al. (2017). Evidence for overuse of medical services around the world. *The Lancet*, 390(10090), 156–68.

Buchan, J., Dhillon, I. S. and Campbell, J. (eds.) (2017). *Health Employment and Economic Growth: An Evidence Base*. Geneva: World Health Organization.

Buchanan, J. M. (1975a). *The Samaritan's dilemma*. In E. S. Phelps (ed.), *Altruism, Morality and Economic Theory*. New York: Russell Sage foundation, pp. 71–85.

Buchanan, J. M. (1975b). *The Limits of Liberty: Between Anarchy and Leviathan*. Chicago: University of Chicago Press.

Buchanan, J. M. (1986). The Constitution of Economic Policy, Nobel Prize lecture. Republished in 1987 in *American Economic Review*, 77(3), 243–50.

Buchanan, J. M. and Tullock, G. (1962). *The Calculus of Consent* (Vol. 3). Ann Arbor: University of Michigan Press.

Buse, K. and Walt, G. (2000). Global public-private partnerships: Part I – A new development in health? *Bulletin of the World Health Organization*, 78, 549–61.

Cameron, D. R. (1978). The expansion of the public economy: A comparative analysis. *The American Political Science Review*, 72(4), 1243–61.

Carapinha, J. L., Ross-Degnan, D., Desta, A. T. and Wagner, A. K. (2011). Health insurance systems in five Sub-Saharan African countries: Medicine benefits and data for decision making. *Health Policy*, 99(3), 193–202.

Carpenter, D. and Moss, D. (2013). *Preventing Regulatory Capture: Special Interest Influence and How to Limit It*. New York: Cambridge University Press.

Carpenter, D. P., Esterling, K. M. and Lazer, D. M. (1998). The strength of weak ties in lobbying networks: Evidence from health-care politics in the United States. *Journal of Theoretical Politics*, 10(4), 417–44.

Casalino, L. P., Nicholson, S., Gans, D. N. et al. (2009). What does it cost physician practices to interact with health insurance plans? *Health Affairs*, 28, w533–43.

Casamatta, G., Cremer, H. and Pestieau, P. (2000). Political sustainability and the design of social insurance. *Journal of Public Economics*, 75(3), 341–64.

Case, A. and Deaton, A. (2015). Rising morbidity and mortality in midlife among white non-Hispanic Americans in the 21st century. *Proceedings of the National Academy of Sciences*, 112(49), 15078–83.

Caudill, S. B., Ford, J. M. and Kaserman, D. L. (1995). Certificate-of-need regulation and the diffusion of innovation: A random coefficient model. *Journal of Applied Econometrics*, 10, 73–8.

Chadavarkar, R. (1992). Plague panic and epidemic politics in India, 1896–1914. In T. Ranger and P. Slack (eds.), *Epidemics and Ideas: Essays on the Historical Perception of Pestilence*. Cambridge: Cambridge University Press, pp. 101–24.

Chalkley, M. and Malcomson, J. M. (1998). Contracting for health services when patient demand does not reflect quality. *Journal of Health Economics*, 17(1), 1–19.

Chandra, A. and Skinner, J. (2012). Technology growth and expenditure growth in health care. *Journal of Economic Literature*, 50(3), 645–80.

Chandra, A. and Staiger, D. O. (2017). Identifying sources of inefficiency in health care. NBER Working Paper No. 24035.

Chattopadhyay, R. and Duflo, E. (2004). Women and policy makers: Evidence from a randomised policy experiment in India. *Econometrica*, 72(5), 1409–43.

Chaudhury, N., Hammer, J., Kremer, M., Muralidharan, K. and Rogers, F. H. (2006). Missing in action: Teacher and health worker absence in developing countries. *Journal of Economic Perspectives*, 20(1), 91–116.

Chen, A. and Goldman, D. (2016). Health care spending: Historical trends and new directions. *Annual Review of Economics*, 8, 291–319.

Chernew, M. E. and Newhouse, J. P. (2012). Health care spending growth. In M. V. Pauly, T. G. McGuire and P. P. Barros (eds.), *Handbook of Health Economics* (Vol. 2). London: North Holland, pp. 1–38.

Congleton, R. D. (2003). The median voter model. In C. K. Rowley and F. Schneider (eds.) *The Encyclopedia of Public Choice*. Boston, MA: Springer, pp. 707–12.

Congleton, R. and Bose, F. (2010). The rise of the modern welfare state, ideology, institutions, and income security: Analysis and evidence. *Public Choice*, 144, 535–55.

Congleton, R. D., Batinti, A., Bose, F., Kim, Y. and Pietrantonio, R. (2011). Public choice and the modern welfare state, on the growth of government in the twentieth century. In M. Reksulak, L. Razzolini and W. F. Shughart (eds.), *Elgar Companion to Public Choice*, 2nd edn. Cheltenham: Edward Elgar, pp. 362–81.

Congleton, R. D., Batinti, A. and Pietrantonio, R. (2017). The electoral politics and the evolution of complex healthcare systems. *Kyklos*, 70(4), 483–510.

Conrad, P. (2007). *The Medicalization of Society: On the Transformation of Human Conditions into Treatable Disorders*. Baltimore: Johns Hopkins University Press.

Cooper, Z., Kowalski, A. E., Powell, E. N. and Wu, J. (2017). Politics, hospital behavior, and health care spending. NBER Working Paper No. 23748.

Coretti, S., Costa-Font, J., Rodon, T. and Turati, G. (2020). Do medical doctors make better health ministers? Unpublished Working Paper.

Cornia, G. (2001). Globalization and health: Results and options. *Bulletin of the World Health Organization*, 79(9), 843–41.

Couffinhal, A. and Socha-Dietrich, K. (2017). Ineffective spending and waste in health care systems: Framework and findings. In OECD, *Tackling Wasteful Spending in Health*. Paris: OECD Publishing, pp. 17–59.

Costa-Font, J. (2009). Simultaneity, asymmetric devolution and economic incentives in Spanish regional elections. *Regional and Federal Studies*, 19(1), 165–84.

Costa-Font, J. (2010a). Devolution, diversity and welfare reform: Long-term care in the 'Latin Rim'. *Social Policy & Administration*, 44(4), 481–94.

Costa-Font, J. (2010b). Does devolution lead to regional inequalities in welfare activity? *Environment and Planning C: Government and Policy*, 28(3), 435–49.

Costa-Font, J. (2016). Deregulation and access to medicines: The Peruvian experience. *Journal of International Development*, 28(6), 997–1005.

Costa-Font, J. and Cowell, F. (2019). Incorporating inequality aversion in healthcare priority setting. *Social Justice Research*, 32(2), 172–85.

Costa-Font, J. and Ferrer-i Carbonell, A. (2019). Regional decentralisation and the demand for public health care. FEDEA Working Paper.

Costa-Font, J. and Garcia, J. (2003). Demand for private health insurance: How important is the quality gap? *Health Economics*, 12(7), 587–99.

Costa-Font, J. and Greer, S. (2013). *Federalism and Decentralization in European Health and Social Care*. Basingstoke: Palgrave Macmillan.

Costa-Font, J. and Jofre-Bonet, M. (2008). Is there a 'secession of the wealthy'? Private health insurance uptake and National Health System support. *Bulletin of Economic Research*, 60(3), 265–87.

Costa-Font, J. and Mas, N. (2016). 'Globesity'? The effects of globalization on obesity and caloric intake. *Food Policy*, 64, 121–32.

Costa-Font, J. and Moscone, F. (2008). The impact of decentralization and inter-territorial interactions on Spanish health expenditure. *Empirical Economics*, 34(1), 167–84.

Costa-Font, J. and Pons-Novell, J. (2007). Public health expenditure and spatial interactions in a decentralized national health system. *Health Economics*, 16(3), 291–306.

Costa-Font, J. and Puig-Junoy, J. (2007). Institutional change, innovation and regulation failure: Evidence from the Spanish drug market. *Policy and Politics*, 35(4), 701–18.

Costa-Font, J. and Rico, A. (2006a). Vertical competition in the Spanish National Health System (NHS). *Public Choice*, 128(3–4), 477–98.

Costa-Font, J. and Rico, A. (2006b). Devolution and the interregional inequalities in health and healthcare in Spain. *Regional Studies*, 40(8), 1–13.

Costa-Font, J. and Turati, G. (2018). Regional healthcare decentralization in unitary states: Equal spending, equal satisfaction? *Regional Studies*, 52(7), 974–85.

Costa-Font, J. and Zigante, V. (2016). The choice agenda in European health systems: The role of middle-class demands. *Public Money & Management*, 36(6), 409–16.

Costa-Font, J., Gemmill, M. and Rubert, G. (2011a). Biases in the healthcare luxury good hypothesis?: A meta-regression analysis. *Journal of the Royal Statistical Society: Series A (Statistics in Society)*, 174(1), 95–107.

Costa-Font, J., Salvador-Carulla, L., Cabases, J., Alonso, J. and McDaid, D. (2011b). Tackling neglect and mental health reform in a devolved system of welfare governance. *Journal of Social Policy*, 40, 295–312.

Costa-Font, J., McGuire, A. and Serra-Sastre, V. (2012). The 'Weisbrod quadri-lemma' revisited: Insurance incentives on new health technologies. *The Geneva Papers on Risk and Insurance – Issues and Practice*, 37(4), 678–95.

Costa-Font, J., Jofre-Bonet, M. and Yen, S. T. (2013). Not all incentives wash out the warm glow: The case of blood donation revisited. *Kyklos*, 66(4), 529–51.

Costa-Font, J., De-Albuquerque, F. and Doucouliagos, H. (2014). Do jurisdictions compete on taxes? A meta-regression analysis. *Public Choice*, 161(3–4), 451–70.

Costa-Font, J., Hernandez-Quevedo, C. and Sato, A. (2018). A health 'Kuznets curve'? Cross-sectional and longitudinal evidence on concentration indices. *Social Indicators Research*, 136(2), 439–52.

Crivelli, E., Leive, A. and Stratmann, T. (2010). Subnational health spending and soft budget constraints in OECD countries. IMF Working Paper No. 10/147.

Cutler, D. M. (2007). The lifetime costs and benefits of medical technology. *Journal of Health Economics*, 26, 1081–100.

Cutler, D. M. and Johnson, R. (2004). The birth and growth of the social insurance state: Explaining old age and medical insurance across countries. *Public Choice*, 120(1–2), 87–121.

Cutler, D. M. and McClellan, M. (2001). Is technological change in medicine worth it? *Health Affairs*, 20(5), 11–29.

Cutler, D. M., Wickler, E. and Basch, P. (2012). Reducing administrative costs and improving the health care system. *New England Journal of Medicine*, 367(20), 1875–8.

Dahl, R. A. (1971). *Polyarchy: Participation and Opposition*. New Haven, CT: Yale University Press.

Dal Bó, E. (2006). Regulatory capture: A review. *Oxford Review of Economic Policy*, 22(2), 203–25.

De Donder, P. and Hindriks, J. (2007). Equilibrium social insurance with policy-motivated parties. *European Journal of Political Economy*, 23(3), 624–40.

Deaton, A. (2002). Policy implications of the gradient of health and wealth. *Health Affairs*, 21(2), 13–30.

Deaton, A. S. (2004). Health in an age of globalization. In S. M. Collins and C. Graham (eds.), *Brookings Trade Forum*. Washington, DC: Brookings Institution Press, pp. 83–130.

Deaton, A. (2014). The Great Escape: Health, Wealth and the Origins of Inequality, Princeton University Press.

Delipalla, S. and O'Donnell, O. (1999).The political economy of a publicly provided private good with adverse selection. Department of Economics Discussion Paper No. 9911, University of Kent.

DellaVigna, S. and Kaplan, E. (2007). The Fox News effect: Media bias and voting. *The Quarterly Journal of Economics*, 122(3), 1187–234.

Downs, A. (1957a). An economic theory of political action in a democracy. *Journal of Political Economy*, 65(2), 135–50.

Downs, A. (1957b). *An Economic Theory of Democracy*. New York: Harper & Row.

Dror, D. M., Hossain, S. A. S., Majumdar, A., Pérez Koehlmoos, T. L., John, D. and Panda, P. K. (2016). What factors affect voluntary uptake of community-based health insurance schemes in low- and middle-income countries? A systematic review and meta-analysis. *PLoS ONE*, 11(8), e0160479. https://doi.org/10.1371/journal.pone.0160479.

Dulleck, U. and Kerschbamer, R. (2006). On doctors, mechanics and computer specialists: The economics of credence goods. *Journal of Economic Literature*, 44(1), 5–42.

Durante, R., Pinotti, P. and Tesei, A. (2019). The political legacy of entertainment TV. *American Economic Review*, 109(7), 2497–530.

Dustmann, C., Vasiljeva, K. and Damm, A. P. (2019). Refugee migration and electoral outcomes. *Review of Economic Studies*, 86(5), 2035–91.

Dybczak, K. and Przywara, B. (2010). The role of technology in health care expenditure in the EU. European Commission Economic Paper No. 400.

Easterly, W. and Levine, R. (1997). Africa's growth tragedy: Policies and ethnic divisions. *Quarterly Journal of Economics*, 112, 1203–50.

Eddy, D. M. (1984). Variations in physician practice: The role of uncertainty. *Health Affairs*, 3(2), 74–89.

Elster, J. (1994). The impact of constitutions on economic performance. *The World Bank Economic Review*, 8(1), 209–26.

Epple, D. and Romano, R. E. (1996a). Ends against the middle: Determining public service provision when there are private alternatives. *Journal of Public Economics*, 62, 297–325.

Epple, D. and Romano, R. E. (1996b). Public provision of private goods. *Journal of Political Economy*, 104, 57–84.

European Commission. (2007). White Paper 'Together for health: A strategic approach for the EU 2008–2013', COM(2007) 630 final, Brussels, 23 October.

Fabbri, D. and Robone, S. (2010). The geography of hospital admission in a national health service with patient choice. *Health Economics*, 19, 1029–47.

Fidler, D. P. (2010). The challenges of global health governance. Council on Foreign Relations, International Institutions and Global Governance Program Working Paper, May.

Francese, M., Piacenza, M., Romanelli, M. and Turati, G. (2014). Understanding inappropriateness in health spending: The role of regional policies and institutions in caesarean deliveries. *Regional Science and Urban Economics*, 49(C), 262–77.

Franco, A., Alvarez-Darde, C. and Ruiz, M. (2004). Effect of democracy on health: Ecological study. *British Medical Journal*, 329, 1421–3.

Frandsen, B. R., Joynt, K. E., Rebitzer, J. B. and Jha, A. K. (2015). Care fragmentation, quality, and costs among chronically ill patients. *The American Journal of Managed Care*, 21(5), 355–62.

Frey, B. S. and Stutzer, A. (2000). Happiness prospers in democracy. *Journal of Happiness Studies*, 1(1), 79–102.

Frey, R. and Al-Roumi, A. (1999). Political democracy and the physical quality of life: The cross-national evidence. *Social Indicators Research*, 47, 73–97.

Fried, H., Lovell, K. and Schmidt, S. (2007). *The Measurement of Productive Efficiency and Productivity*. Oxford: Oxford University Press.

Gamkhar, S. and Shah, A. (2007). The impact of intergovernmental fiscal transfers: A synthesis of the conceptual and empirical literature. In R. Boadway and A. Shah (eds.), *Intergovernmental Fiscal Transfers: Principles and Practice*. Washington, DC: World Bank, pp. 225–58.

Gans, J. S. and Smart, M. (1996). Majority voting with single-crossing preferences. *Journal of Public Economics*, 59, 219–37.

Gao, Y., Zang, L., Roth, A. and Wang, P. (2017). Does democracy cause innovation? An empirical test of the popper hypothesis. *Research Policy*, 46(7), 1272–83.

Garber, A. M. and Skinner, J. (2008). Is American health care uniquely inefficient? *Journal of Economic Perspectives*, 22(4), 27–50.

Gerring, J., Thacker, S. C. and Alfaro, R. (2012). Democracy and human development. *The Journal of Politics*, 74(1), 1–17.

Ghobarah, H. A., Huth, P. and Russett, B. (2004a). Comparative public health: The political economy of human misery and well-being. *International Studies Quarterly*, 48(1), 73–94.

Ghobarah, H. A., Huth, P. and Russett, B. (2004b). The post-war public health effects of civil conflict. *Social Science & Medicine*, 59(4), 869–84.

Godefroy, R. (2011). The birth of the congressional clinic. PSE Working Papers No. 00564921.

Goodin, R. E. and Le Grand, J. (1987). *Not Only the Poor: The Middle Classes and the Welfare State*. London: Taylor & Francis.

Goodspeed, T. J. (2002). Tax competition and tax structure in open federal economies: Evidence from OECD countries with implications for the European Union. *European Economic Review*, 46(2), 357–74.

Gottschalk, F., Mimra, W. and Waibel, C. (2018). Health services as credence goods: A field experiment (25 July). Available at SSRN: https://ssrn.com/abstract=3036573 or http://dx.doi.org/10.2139/ssrn.3036573.

Gouveia, M. (1997). Majority rule and the public provision of a private good. *Public Choice*, 93, 221–44.

Greer, S. L. (2008). Choosing paths in European Union health services policy: A political analysis of a critical juncture. *Journal of European Social Policy*, 18(3), 219–31.

Greer, S. L. and Méndez, C. A. (2015). Universal health coverage: A political struggle and governance challenge. *American Journal of Public Health*, 105 (Suppl 5), S637–9. http://doi.org/10.2105/AJPH.2015.302733.

Grossman, G. M. and Helpman, E. (2001). *Special Interest Politics*. Cambridge, MA: MIT Press.

Grossman, M. (1972a). *The Demand for Health: A Theoretical and Empirical Investigation*. New York: NBER Books.

Grossman, M. (1972b). On the concept of health capital and the demand for health. *Journal of Political Economy*, 80(2), 223–55.

Gründler, K. and Krieger, T. (2018). Machine learning indices, political institutions, and economic development. CESifo Working Paper No. 6930, CESifo Group Munich.

Gutschoven, K. and van den Bulck, J. (2004). Television viewing and smoking volume in adolescent smokers: A cross-sectional study. *Preventive Medicine*, 39(6), 1093–8.

Hale, T., Held, D. and Young, K. (2013). *Gridlock: Why Multilateral Cooperation Is Failing When We Need It Most*. Cambridge: Polity.

Hall, R. E. and Jones, C. I. (2007). The value of life and the rise in health spending. *The Quarterly Journal of Economics*, 122(1), 39–72.

Hall, R. L. and Deardorff, A. V. (2006). Lobbying as legislative subsidy. *American Political Science Review*, 100, 169–84.

Hanna, K., Röth, L. and Garritzmann, J. L. (2018). Ideological alignment and the distribution of public expenditures. *West European Politics*, 41(3), 779–802.

Hayek, F. A. (1948). *Individualism and Economic Order*. Chicago: University of Chicago Press.

Hegde, D. (2009). Political influence behind the veil of peer review: An analysis of public biomedical research funding in the United States. *The Journal of Law and Economics*, 52(4), 665–90.

Hegde, D. and Mowery, D. (2008). Politics and funding in the U.S. public biomedical R&D system. *Science*, 322(5909), 1797–8.

Hegde, D. and Sampat, B. (2015). Can private money buy public science? Disease group lobbying and federal funding for biomedical research. *Management Science*, 61(10), 2281–98.

Hindriks, J. and De Donder, P. (2003). The politics of redistributive social insurance. *Journal of Public Economics*, 87(12), 2639–60.

Hines, J. R. and Thaler, R. H. (1995). The flypaper effect. *Journal of Economic Perspectives*, 9(4), 217–26.

Hogan, D. R., Stevens, G. A., Hosseinpoor, A. R. and Boerma, T. (2018). Monitoring universal health coverage within the Sustainable Development Goals: Development and baseline data for an index of essential health services. *The Lancet – Global Health*, 6(2), e152–68. https://doi.org/10.1016/S2214-109X(17)30472-2.

Holcombe, R. G. (1989). The median voter model in public choice theory. *Public Choice*, 61, 115–25.

Hollingsworth, B. (2008). The measurement of efficiency and productivity of health care delivery. *Health Economics*, 17(10), 1107–28.

Hollingsworth, B. and Peacock, S. J. (2008). *Efficiency Measurement in Health and Health Care*. London: Taylor & Francis.

Holmberg, S. and Rothstein, B. (2011). Dying of corruption. *Health Economics, Policy and Law*, 6, 529–47.

Horowitz, M. D., Rosensweig, J. A. and Jones, C. A. (2007). Medical tourism: Globalization of healthcare marketplace. *Medscape General Medicine*, 9(4), 33–41.

Horwitz, J. R. (2007). Does nonprofit ownership matter? *Yale Journal on Regulation*, 24(1), 139–204.

Hotelling, H. (1929). Stability in competition. *Economic Journal*, 39, 41–57.

House of Commons. (2011). House of Commons Treasury Committee. Private finance initiative. 17th report of session 2010–12.

Houweling, T. A., Kunst, A. E., Looman, C. W. and Mackenbach, J. P. (2005). Determinants of under-5 mortality among the poor and the rich: A cross-national analysis of 43 developing countries. *International Journal of Epidemiology*, 34(6), 1257–65.

Hsia, R. Y., Akosa Antwi, Y. and Weber, E. (2014). Analysis of variation in charges and prices paid for vaginal and caesarean section births: A cross-sectional study. *BMJ Open*, 4(1), e004017.

Hussey, P. S., De Vries, H., Romley, J. et al. (2009). A systematic review of health care efficiency measures. *Health Services Research*, 44(3), 784–805.

Iliffe, J. (1995). *Africans: The History of a Continent*. Cambridge: Cambridge University Press.

Inglehart, R., Foa, R., Peterson, C. and Welzel, C. (2008). Development, freedom, and rising happiness: A global perspective (1981–2007). *Perspectives on Psychological Science*, 3(4), 264–85.

Iqbal, Z. (2006). Health and human security: The public health impact of violent conflict. *International Studies Quarterly*, 50, 631–49.

Jacob, J. and Lundin, D. (2005). A median voter model of health insurance with ex post moral hazard. *Journal of Health Economics*, 24(2), 407–26.

Jaffe, S. (2015). USA grapples with high drug costs. *The Lancet*, 386, 2127–8.

Kaitelidou, D., Tsirona, C. S., Galanis, P. A. et al. (2013). Informal payments for maternity health services in public hospitals in Greece. *Health Policy*, 109(1), 23–30. https://doi.org/10.1016/j.healthpol.2012.10.012.

Kelly, C., Tumblety, J. and Sheron, N. (2016). Histories of medical lobbying. *The Lancet*, 388(10055), 1976–7.

Kifmann, M. (2005). Health insurance in a democracy: Why is it public and why are premiums income-related? *Public Choice*, 124, 283–308.

Kifmann, M. (2009). Political economy of healthcare. In P. Zweifel, F. Breyer and M. Kifmann (eds.), *Health Economics*. New York: Springer Science & Business Media, pp. 429–46.

Kifmann, M. and Roeder, K. (2018). The political sustainability of a basic income scheme and social health insurance. *Journal of Public Economic Theory*, 1–20.

Kleider, H., Röth, L. and Garritzmann, J. L. (2018). Ideological alignment and the distribution of public expenditures. *West European Politics*, 41(3), 779–802.

Klomp, J. and De Haan, J. (2009). Is the political system really related to health? *Social Science & Medicine*, 69(1), 36–46.

Koethenbuerger, M. (2008). Revisiting the 'decentralization theorem': On the role of externalities. *Journal of Urban Economics*, 64, 116–22.

Kotakorpi, K. and Laamanen, J.-P. (2010). Welfare state and life satisfaction: Evidence from public health care. *Economica*, 77(307), 565–83.

Krueger, A. (1974). The political economy of the rent-seeking society. *American Economic Review*, 64, 291–303.

Krueger, P. M., Dovel, K. and Denney, J. T. (2015). Democracy and self-rated health across 67 countries: A multilevel analysis. *Social Science and Medicine*, 143, 137–44.

Kudamatsu, M. (2012). Has democratization reduced infant mortality in sub-Saharan Africa? Evidence from micro data. *Journal of the European Economic Association*, 10(6), 1294–1317.

Kumbhakar, S. C. and Knox Lovell, C. A. (2000). *Stochastic Frontier Analysis*. Cambridge: Cambridge University Press.

Kushel, M. and Bindman, A. B. (2004). Health care lobbying: Time to make patients the special interest. *The American Journal of Medicine*, 116(7), 496–7.

Kwak, J. (2013). Cultural capture and the financial crisis. In D. Carpenter and D. Moss (eds.), *Preventing Regulatory Capture: Special Interest Influence and How to Limit It*. New York: Cambridge University Press, pp. 71–98.

La Ferrara, E., Chong, A. and Duryea, S. (2012). Soap operas and fertility: Evidence from Brazil. *American Economic Journal: Applied Economics*, 4(4), 1–31.

Labelle, R., Stoddart, G. and Rice, T. (1994). A re-examination of the meaning and importance of supplier induced demand. *Journal of Health Economics*, 13, 347–68.

Laffont, J. J. (2000). *Incentives and Political Economy*. Oxford: Oxford University Press.

Landers, S. H. and Sehgal, A. R. (2000). How do physicians lobby their members of Congress? *Archives of Internal Medicine*, 160(21), 3248–51.

Landers, S. H. and Sehgal, A. R. (2004). Health care lobbying in the United States. *The American Journal of Medicine*, 116(7), 474–7.

Le Grand, J. (1991). The theory of government failure. *British Journal of Political Science*, 21(4), 423–42.

Le Grand, J. (2002). The labour government and the National Health Service. *Oxford Review of Economic Policy*, 18(2), 137–53.

Le Moglie, M. and Turati, G. (2019). Electoral cycle bias in the media coverage of corruption news. *Journal of Economic Behavior and Organization*, 163(C), 140–57.

Leaver, C. (2009). Bureaucratic minimal squawk behaviour: Theory and evidence from regulatory agencies. *American Economic Review*, 99(3), 572–607.

Lena, H. and London, B. (1993). The political and economic determinants of health outcomes: A cross-national analysis. *International Journal of Health Services*, 23, 585–602.

Levaggi, R. and Zanola, R. (2007). Patients' migration across regions: The case of Italy. *Applied Economics*, 36(16), 1751–7.

Levy, G. (2005). The politics of public provision of education. *The Quarterly Journal of Economics*, 120(4), 1507–34.

Li, Q. and Wen, M. (2005). The immediate and lingering effects of armed conflict on adult mortality: A time-series cross-national analysis. *Journal of Peace Research*, 42, 471–92.

Li, S. M., Moslehi, S. and Yew, S. L. (2016). Public–private mix of health expenditure: A political economy and quantitative analysis. Canadian Journal of Economics/*Revue canadienne d'économique*, 49(2), 834–66.

Lichtenberg, F. R. and Virabhak, S. (2002). Pharmaceutical-embodied technical progress, longevity, and quality of life: Drugs as 'equipment for your health'. NBER Working Paper No. 9351.

Lipset, S. M. (1959). Some social requisites of democracy: Economic development and political legitimacy. *American Political Science Review*, 53(1), 69–105.

López-Casasnovas, G., Costa-Font, J. and Planas, I. (2005). Diversity and regional inequalities in the Spanish system of health care services. *Health Economics*, 14(S1), 221–35.

Loubser, R. and Steenekamp, C. (2017). Democracy, well-being, and happiness: A 10-nation study. *Journal of Public Affairs*, 17(1–2), e1646.

Lyu, H., Xu, T., Brotman, D. et al. (2017). Overtreatment in the United States. *PLoS One*, 12(9), e0181970.

Mackenbach, J. P. and McKee, M. (2013). Social-democratic government and health policy in Europe: A quantitative analysis. *International Journal of Health Services*, 43(3), 389–41.

Maisonneuve, C., Moreno-Serra, R., Murtin, F. and Oliveira Martins, J. (2017). The role of policy and institutions on health spending. *Health Economics*, 26(7), 834–43.

Makkai, T. and Braithwaite, J. (1992). In and out of the revolving door: Making sense of regulatory capture. *Journal of Public Policy*, 12(1), 61–78.

Mann, J. M., Gostin, L., Gruskin, S., Brennan, T., Lazzarini, Z. and Fineberg, H. V. (1994). Health and human rights. *Health and Human Rights*, 1, 6–23.

Marchildon, G. P. and Bossert, T. J. (2018). Federalism and decentralization in the health care sector. Forum of Federations Occasional Paper No. 24.

Margolis, H. (1984). *Selfishness, Altruism, and Rationality*. Chicago: University of Chicago Press.

Markides, K. S. (1983). Mortality among minority populations: A review of recent patterns and trends. *Public Health Reports*, 98(3), 252–60.

Matesanz, R. (1996). The panorama effect on altruistic organ donation. *Transplantation*, 62(11), 1700–1.

Mathers, C. D. and Loncar, D. (2006). Projections of global mortality and burden of disease from 2002 to 2030. *PLoS Medicine*, 3(11), e442.

Matsuura, H. (2012). Rights, health laws, and health outcomes. Sc. D. dissertation, Harvard University.

Matsuura, H. (2013). The effect of a constitutional right to health on population health in 157 countries, 1970–2007: The role of democratic governance. PGDA Working Paper No. 106, Harvard University.

Matsuura, H. (2014). Does the constitutional right to health matter? A review of current evidence. *CESifo DICE Report*, 12(2), 35–41.

McDonough, J. E. (2012). *Inside National Health Reform*. Berkeley: University of California Press.

McGuire, J. W. (2006). Democracy, basic service utilization, and under-5 mortality: A cross-national study of developing states. *World Development*, 34(3), 405–25.

McGuire, J. W. (2010). *Wealth, Health, and Democracy in East Asia and Latin America*. Cambridge: Cambridge University Press.

McIntyre, D., Rogers, L. and Heier, E. J. (2001). Overview, history, and objectives of performance measurement. *Health Care Financing Review*, 22(3), 7–21.

Mehrortra, S. (2006). Governance and basic social services: Ensuring accountability in service delivery through deep democratic decentralisation. *Journal of International Development*, 18, 263–83.

Meltzer, A. H. and Richard, S. F. (1981). A rational theory of the size of government. *Journal of Political Economy*, 89(5), 914–27.

Merlo, A. (2006). Whither political economy? Theories, facts and issues. In R. Blundell, W. K. Newey and T. Persson (eds.), *Advances in Economics and Econometrics: Theory and Applications, Ninth World Congress* (Vol. I, No. 41). Cambridge: Cambridge University Press, pp. 381–421.

Mestres, A. J., López-Casasnovas, G. and Castelló, J. V. (2018). The deadly effects of losing health insurance. CRES-UPF Working Paper No. 201804-104.

Milanovic, B. (2000). The median-voter hypothesis, income inequality, and income redistribution: An empirical test with the required data. *European Journal of Political Economy*, 16(3), 367–410.

Miljkovic, D., Shaik, S., Miranda, S., Barabanov, N. and Liogier, A. (2015). Globalisation and obesity. *World Economy*, 38(8), 1278–94.

Miller, G. (2008). Women's suffrage, political responsiveness, and child survival in American history. *Quarterly Journal of Economics*, 123(3), 1287–132.

Mobarak, A. M., Rajkumar, A. S. and Cropper, M. (2011). The political economy of health services provision in Brazil. *Economic Development and Cultural Change*, 59(4), 723–51.

Moe, T. (1987). An assessment of the positive theory of 'congressional dominance'. *Legislative Studies Quarterly*, 12, 475–520.

Moe, T. M. and Wilson, S. A. (1994). Presidents and the politics of structure. *Law and Contemporary Problems*, 57(2), 1–44.

Moene, K. O. and Wallerstein, M. (2003). Earnings inequality and welfare spending: A disaggregated analysis. *World Politics*, 55, 485–516.

Montolio, D. and Turati, G. (2017). Constitutions as incomplete social contracts. *Politica Economica*, 33(3), 259–68.

Moreno-Ternero, J. and Roemer, J. E. (2010). The political economy of health care finance. CORE Discussion Papers No. 2007031.

Moscone, F., Tosetti, E. and Vittadini, G. (2012). Social interaction in patients' hospital choice: Evidence from Italy. *Journal of the Royal Statistical Society Series A*, 175(2), 453–72.

Mossialos, E. and Thomson, S. (2004). Voluntary health insurance in the European Union. European Observatory on Health Systems and Policies. www.euro.who.int/__data/assets/pdf_file/0006/98448/E84885.pdf.

Mossialos, E., Costa-Font, J., Davaki, K. and Karras, K. (2005). Is there 'patient selection' in the demand for private maternity care in Greece? *Applied Economics Letters*, 12(1), 7–12.

Mueller, D. C. (1976). Public choice: A survey. *Journal of Economic Literature*, 14(2), 395–433.

Mueller, D. C. (2003). *Public Choice III*. Cambridge: Cambridge University Press.

Mulligan, C., Gil, R. and Sala-i-Martin, X. (2004). Do democracies have different public policies than nondemocracies? *Journal of Economic Perspectives*, 18(1), 51–74.

Mulumba, M., Kabanda, D. and Nassuna, V. (2010). Constitutional provisions for the right to health in east and southern Africa. Centre for Health, Human Rights and Development (CEHURD) in the Regional Network for Equity in Health in East and Southern Africa. EQUINET Discussion Paper No. 81, April.

Muntaner, C., Borrell, C., Ng, E., Chung, H., Espelt, A., Rodriguez-Sanz, M. and O'Campo, P. (2011). Politics, welfare regimes, and population health: Controversies and evidence. *Sociology of Health & Illness*, 33(6), 946–64.

Murphy, K. M. and Topel, R. H. (2003a). The economic value of medical research. In K. M. Murphy and R. H. Topel (eds.), *Measuring the Gains from Medical Research: An Economic Approach*. Chicago: University of Chicago Press, pp. 9–40.

Murphy, K. M. and Topel, R. H. (eds.). (2003b). *Measuring the Gains from Medical Research: An Economic Approach*. Chicago: University of Chicago Press.

Murphy, K. M. and Topel, R. H. (2006). The value of health and longevity. *Journal of Political Economy*, 114(5), 871–904.

Naci, H., Wouters, O. J., Gupta, R. and Ioannidis, J. P. A. (2017). Timing and characteristics of cumulative evidence available on novel therapeutic agents receiving Food and Drug Administration accelerated approval. *Milbank Quarterly*, 95(2), 261–90.

National Audit Office. (2018). PFI and PF2. www.nao.org.uk/report/pfi-and-pf2/.

Navarro, V., Muntaner, C., Borrell, C. et al. (2006). Politics and health outcomes. *The Lancet*, 368(9540), 1033–7.

Newbold, K. B. (2005). Self-rated health within the Canadian immigrant population: Risk and the healthy immigrant effect. *Social Science and Medicine*, 60(6), 1359–70.

Newhouse, J. P. (1992). Medical care costs: How much welfare loss? *Journal of Economic Perspectives*, 6(3), 3–21.

Niskanen, W. A. (1971). *Bureaucracy and Representative Government*. Chicago: Aldine Atherton.

North, D. (1990a). Institutions and their consequences for economic performance. In K. Schweers Cook and M. Levi (eds.), *The Limits of Rationality*. Chicago: University of Chicago Press, pp. 383–401.

North, D. (1990b). *Institutions, Institutional Change and Economic Performance*. Cambridge: Cambridge University Press.

Nyman, J. A. (2004). Is 'moral hazard' inefficient? The policy implications of a new theory. *Health Affairs*, 23(5), 194–9.

Oates, W. E. (1972). *Fiscal Federalism*. New York: Harcourt, Brace, Jovanovich.

Oates, W. E. (1985). Searching for the Leviathan: An empirical study. *American Economic Review*, 75(4), 748–57.

Oates, W. E. (1999). An essay on fiscal federalism. *American Economic Review*, 37(3), 1120–49.

Obama, B. (2016). United States health care reform: Progress to date and next steps. *JAMA*, 316(5), 525–32.

OECD. (2009). Explaining the sub-national tax-grants balance in OECD countries. OECD Network on Fiscal Relations across Levels of Government. Paris: OECD Publishing.

OECD. (2016). *Fiscal Federalism 2016: Making Decentralisation Work*. Paris: OECD Publishing.

OECD. (2018). Preventing policy capture: Integrity in public decision-making. OECD Public Governance Reviews. Paris: OECD Publishing. https://dx.doi.org/10.1787/9789264065239-en.

Okun, A. (1975). *Equality and Efficiency: The Big Trade-Off*. Washington, DC: The Brookings Institute.

Okunade, A. and Murthy, V. (2002). Technology as a 'major driver' of health care costs: A cointegration analysis of the Newhouse conjecture. *Journal of Health Economics*, 21, 147–59.

Olson, M. (1965). *The Logic of Collective Action*. Cambridge, MA: Harvard University Press.

Olson, M. (1982). *The Rise and Decline of Nations: Economic Growth, Stagflation, and Social Rigidities*. New Haven, CT: Yale University Press.

Osewe, P. L. (2017). Options for financing pandemic preparedness. *Bulletin of the World Health Organization*, 95(12), 794.

Oswald, M. (2013). In a democracy, what should a healthcare system do? A dilemma for public policymakers. *Politics, Philosophy & Economics*, 14(1), 23–52.

Padovano, F. (2013). Are we witnessing a paradigm shift in the analysis of political competition? *Public Choice*, 156(3–4), 631–51.

Peltzman, S. (1976). Toward a more general theory of regulation. *The Journal of Law and Economics*, 19(2), 211–40.

Persson, T. and Tabellini, G. (2000). *Political Economics: Explaining Economic Policy*. Cambridge, MA: MIT Press.

Persson, T. and Tabellini, G. (2003). *Economic Effects of Constitutions*. Cambridge, MA: MIT Press.

Persson, T. and Tabellini, G. (2004). Constitutions and economic policy. *Journal of Economic Perspectives*, 18(1), 75–98.

Perucca, G., Piacenza, M. and Turati, G. (2019). Spatial inequality in access to healthcare: Evidence from an Italian Alpine region. *Regional Studies*, 53(4), 478–89.

Pieters, H., Curzi, D., Olper, A. and Swinnen, J. (2016). Effect of democratic reforms on child mortality: A synthetic control analysis. *The Lancet Global Health*, 4(9), e627–32.

Pilny, A. and Roesel, F. (2017). Are doctors better health ministers? The limits of technocracy. Unpublished manuscript, RWI-Essen.

Piperno, S. (2000). Fiscal Decentralisation in Italy: Some Lessons. Mimeo. www.imf .org/external/pubs/ft/seminar/2000/idn/italy.pdf.

Plott, C. R. (1967). A notion of equilibrium and its possibility under majority rule. *The American Economic Review*, 57(4), 787–806.

Posner, R. A. (1974). Theories of economic regulation. *Bell Journal of Economics and Management Science*, 5(335), 335–58.

Potrafke, N. (2010). The growth of public health expenditures in OECD countries: Do government ideology and electoral motives matter? *Journal of Health Economics*, 29(6), 797–810.

Powell-Jackson, T., Basu, S., Balabanova, D., McKee, M. and Stuckler, D. (2011). Democracy and growth in divided societies: A health-inequality trap? *Social Science and Medicine*, 73, 33–41.

Preston, S. H. (1975). The changing relation between mortality and level of economic development. *Population Studies*, 29(2), 231–48.

Przeworski, A., Alvarez, M. E., Cheibub, J. A. and Limongi, F. (2000). *Democracy and Development: Political Institutions and Well-Being in the World, 1950–1990*. Cambridge: Cambridge University Press.

Pushkar, M. G. (2012). Democracy and infant mortality in India's 'mini-democracies': A preliminary theoretical inquiry and analysis. *Journal of South Asian Development*, 7(2), 109–37.

Pushkar, M. G. (2013). Nation or state? Where should we look to measure democracy's effects on health? *Forum for Development Studies*, 40(2), 217–33.

Reeves, A., McKee, M., Basu, S. and Stuckler, D. (2014). The political economy of austerity and healthcare: Cross-national analysis of expenditure changes in 27 European nations 1995–2011. *Health Policy*, 115(1), 1–8.

Reich, M. R. (1995). The politics of health sector reform in developing countries: Three cases of pharmaceutical policy. *Health Policy*, 32(1–3), 47–77.

Reidpath, D. D. and Allotey, P. (2006). Structure, (governance) and health: An unsolicited response. *BMC International Health and Human Rights*, 6(1), 12.

Roberts, K. W. (1977). Voting over income tax schedules. *Journal of Public Economics*, 8, 329–40.

Romer, T. (1975). Individual welfare, majority voting, and the properties of a linear income tax. *Journal of Public Economics*, 4, 163–85.

Rose, R. (2004). *Learning from Comparative Public Policy: A Practical Guide*. London: Routledge.

Rosecrance, R. (1999). *The Rise of the Virtual State*. New York: Basic Books.

Rosenberg, D. and Shvetsova, O. (2016). Autocratic health versus democratic health: Different outcome variables for health as a factor versus health as a right. In M. Gallego and N. Schofield (eds.), *The Political Economy of Social Choices*. Switzerland: Springer International Publishing, pp. 1–20.

Ross, M. (2006). Is democracy good for the poor? *American Journal of Political Science*, 50(4), 860–74.

Saez, L. and Sinha, A. (2010). Political cycles, political institutions and public expenditure in India, 1980–2000. *British Journal of Political Science*, 40(1), 91–113.

Safaei, J. (2006). Is democracy good for health? *International Journal of Health Services*, 36, 767–86.

Salmon, P. (1987). Decentralisation as an incentive scheme. *Oxford Review of Economic Policy*, 3(2), 24–43.

Salmon, P. (2019). *Yardstick Competition among Governments: Accountability and Policymaking When Citizens Look across Borders*. Oxford: Oxford University Press.

Sampat, B. (2012). Mission-oriented biomedical research at the NIH. *Research Policy*, 41(10), 1729–41.

Sampat, B., Buterbaugh, K. and Perl, M. (2013). New evidence on the allocation of NIH funds across disease areas. *Milbank Quarterly*, 91(1), 163–85.

Sandler, T. (2004). *Global Collective Action*. Cambridge: Cambridge University Press.

Sangrigoli, A., Sorrenti, G. and Turati, G. (2018). Corruption, mass media, and medical staff behavior: The case of organ donation. Mimeo, University of Zurich.

Savedoff, W. D. and Hussmann, K. (2006). The causes of corruption in the health sector: A focus on health care systems. In Transparency International, *Global Corruption Report 2006: Corruption and Health*. Ann Arbor, MI: Pluto Press, pp. 4–14.

Scervini, F. (2012). Empirics of the median voter: Democracy, redistribution and the role of the middle class. *The Journal of Economic Inequality*, 10(4), 529–50.

Scharpf, F. W. (2002). The European social model. *JCMS: Journal of Common Market Studies*, 40(4), 645–70.

Schmidt, M. G. (1999). Warum die Gesundheitsausgaben wachsen. Befunde des Vergleichs demokratisch verfasster Länder. *Politische Vierteljahresschrift*, 40(2), 229–45.

Schumpeter, J. (1943). *Capitalism, Socialism and Democracy*. London: Unwin.

Seabright, P. (1996). Accountability and decentralisation in government: An incomplete contracts model. *European Economic Review*, 40, 61–9.

Segouin, C., Hodges, B. and Brechat, P. H. (2005). Globalization in health care: Is international standardization of quality a step toward outsourcing? *International Journal for Quality in Health Care*, 17, 277–9.

Shandra, J. M., Nobles, J., London, B. and Williamson, J. B. (2004). Dependency, democracy, and infant mortality: A quantitative, cross-national analysis of less developed countries. *Social Science & Medicine*, 59(2), 321–33.

Shepsle, K. (1979). Institutional arrangements and equilibrium in multidimensional voting models. *American Journal of Political Science*, 23(1), 27–59.

Sheron, N. (2016). Histories of medical lobbying. *The Lancet*, 388(10055), 1976–7.

Shiffman, J. (2007). Has donor prioritization of HIV/AIDS displaced aid for other health issues? *Health Policy and Planning*, 23(2), 95–100.

Shiller, R. J. (2017). Narrative economics. *American Economic Review*, 107(4), 967–1004.

Shkolnikov, V. (1997). The population crisis and rising mortality in transnational Russia. Socioeconomic factors, perceived and self-reported health in Russia: A cross-sectional survey. *Social Science and Medicine*, 47, 269–79.

Shleifer, A. and Vishny, R. W. (1993). Corruption. *The Quarterly Journal of Economics*, 108(3), 599–617.

Silverman, E. and Skinner, J. (2004). Medicare upcoding and hospital ownership. *Journal of Health Economics*, 23(2), 369–89.

Skinner, J. (2011). Causes and consequences of regional variations in health care. In M. Pauly, T. McGuire and P. Barros (eds.), *Handbook of Health Economics* (Vol. 2). Amsterdam: Elsevier, pp. 45–93.

Skinner, J. and Staiger, D. (2015). Technology diffusion and productivity growth in health care. *Review of Economics and Statistics*, 97(5), 951–64.

Smith, R., Beaglehole, R., Woodward, D. and Drager, N. (eds.) (2003). *Global Public Goods for Health: Health Economics and Public Health Perspectives*. Oxford: Oxford University Press.

Smithies, A. (1941). Optimum location in spatial competition. *Journal of Political Economy*, 49(3), 423–39.

Solow, R. M. (1962). Technical progress, capital formation, and economic growth. *The American Economic Review*, 52(2), 76–86.

Sorlie, P. D., Backlund, E., Johnson, N. J. and Rogot, E. (1993). Mortality by Hispanic status in the United States. *JAMA*, 270(20), 2464–8.

Soysa, I. and de Soysa, A. K. (2017). Do globalization & free markets drive obesity among children and youth? An empirical analysis, 1990–2013. *International Interactions*, 44(1), 88–106.

Spithoven, A. (2011). It's the institutions, stupid! Why US health care expenditure is so different from Canada's. *Journal of Economic Issues*, 45(1), 75–96.

Spithoven, A. (2016). The influence of vested interests on healthcare legislation in the USA, 2009–2010. *Journal of Economic Issues*, 50(2), 630–8.

Squires, D. (2014). The global slowdown in health care spending growth. *The Journal of the American Medical Association*, 312, 485–6.

Stegarescu, D. (2005). Public sector decentralisation: Measurement concepts and recent international trends. *Fiscal Studies*, 26(3), 301–3.

Stigler, G. (1957). The tenable range of functions of local government. Federal Expenditure Policy for Economic Growth and Stability. Washington, DC: Joint Economic Committee, Subcommittee on Fiscal Policy, pp. 213–19.

Stigler, G. J. (1971). The theory of economic regulation. *The Bell Journal of Economics and Management Science*, 2(1), 3–21.

Stiglitz, J. E. (1974). The demand for education in public and private school systems. *Journal of Public Economics*, 3, 349–85.

Stiglitz, J. E. (2012). *The Price of Inequality: How Today's Divided Society Endangers Our Future*. New York: W. W. Norton.

Stratmann, T. (2004). Logrolling 1. In C. K. Rowley and F. Schneider (eds.), *The Encyclopedia of Public Choice*. Boston, MA: Springer, pp. 696–9.

Swiss, L., Fallon, K. and Burgos, G. (2012). Reaching a critical mass: Women's political representation and child health in developing countries. *Social Forces*, 91(2), 531–58.

Szucs, T. D., Nichol, K., Meltzer, M., Hak, E., Chancelor, J. and Ammon, C. (2006). Economic and social impact of epidemic and pandemic influenza. *Vaccine*, 24(44–6), 6776–8.

Tabellini, G. (2000). A positive theory of social security. *Scandinavian Journal of Economics*, 102(3), 523–45.

Thomas, L. (1975). *The Lives of a Cell: Notes of a Biology Watcher*. New York: Viking Press.

Thomas, L. (1977). Biomedical science and human health: The long-range prospect. *Daedalus*, 106(3), 163–71.

Thomas, L. (1988). On the science and technology of medicine. *Daedalus*, 117(31), 299–316.

Tiebout, C. M. (1956). A pure theory of local expenditure. *Journal of Political Economy*, 64, 416–42.

Toole, A. A. (2007). Does public scientific research complement private investment in research and development in the pharmaceutical industry? *Journal of Law and Economics*, 50(1), 81–104.

Topel, R. H. (2017). Health economics: A selective historical review for the 125th anniversary of the *Journal of Political Economy*. *Journal of Political Economy*, 125(6), 1868–78.

Transparency International. (2006). *Global Corruption Report 2006: Corruption and Health*. Ann Arbor, MI: Pluto Press.

Tridimas, G. (2001). The economics and politics of the structure of public expenditure. *Public Choice*, 106(3–4), 299–31.

Tsebelis, G. (1995). Decision making in political systems: Veto players in presidentialism, parliamentarism, multicameralism and multipartyism. *British Journal of Political Science*, 25(3), 289–325.

Tsebelis, G. (2002). *Veto Players: How Political Institutions Work*. Princeton, NJ: Princeton University Press.

Tullock, G. (1967). The welfare costs of tariffs, monopolies and theft. *Western Economic Journal*, 5, 224–32.

Tullock, G. (1980). Efficient rent-seeking. In J. Buchanan, R. Tollison and G. Tullock (eds.), *Toward a Theory of the Rent-Seeking Society*. College Station: Texas A&M Press, pp. 97–112.

Tuohy, C. H. and Glied, S. (2013). The political economy of healthcare. In S. Glied and P. C. Smith (eds.), *Oxford Handbook of Health Economics*. Oxford: Oxford University Press, pp. 58–77.

Tuohy, C. H., Flood, C. M. and Stabile, M. (2004). How does private finance affect public health care systems? Marshaling the evidence from OECD nations. *Journal of Health Politics, Policy and Law*, 29(3), 359–96.

Turner, L. (2007). 'First world health care at third world prices': Globalization, bioethics and medical tourism. *BioSocieties*, 2(3), 303–25.

Varkey, P., Kureshi, S. and Lesnick, T. (2010). Empowerment of women and its association with the health of the community. *Journal of Women's Health*, 19(1), 71–6.

Veillard, J., Garcia-Armesto, S., Kadanandale, S. and Klazinga, N. (2009). International health systems comparisons: From measurement challenge to management tool. In P. C. Smith, E. Mossialos, I. Papanicolas and S. Leatherman (eds.), *Performance Measurement for Health Systems Improvement: Experiences, Challenges and Prospects.* Cambridge: Cambridge University Press, pp. 641–72.

Vian, T. (2008). Review of corruption in the health sector: Theory, methods and interventions. *Health Policy and Planning,* 23(2), 83–94.

Vreeland, J. R. (2008). The effect of political regime on civil war: Unpacking anocracy. *Journal of Conflict Resolution,* 52(3), 401–25.

Wahlqvist, M. L. (2006). Weight management in transitional economies: The 'double burden of disease' dilemma. *Asia Pacific Journal of Clinical Nutrition,* 15, 21–9.

Wallis, J. J. and Oates, W. E. (1988). Decentralization in the public sector: An empirical study of state and local government. In H. S. Rosen (ed.), *Fiscal Federalism: Quantitative Studies.* Chicago: University of Chicago Press, pp. 5–32.

Weingast, B. R. and Marshall, W. J. (1988). The industrial organization of Congress: Or, why legislatures, like firms, are not organized as markets. *Journal of Political Economy,* 96, 132–63.

Weingast, B. R. and Wittman, D. A. (2006). The reach of political economy. In B. R. Weingast and D. A. Wittman (eds.), *The Oxford Handbook of Political Economy.* Oxford: Oxford University Press, pp. 3–25.

Weisbrod, B. A. (1991). The health care quadrilemma: An essay on technological change, insurance, quality of care, and cost containment. *Journal of Economic Literature,* 29(2), 523–52.

WHO. (2000). *The World Health Report 2000 – Health Systems: Improving Performance.* Geneva: World Health Organization.

WHO. (2008). Closing the gap in a generation: Health equity through action on the social determinants of health. Commission on the Social Determinants of Health. Geneva: World Health Organization.

WHO. (2010). International migration of health workers. Policy Brief. www.who.int/hrh/resources/oecd-who_policy_brief_en.pdf.

WHO. (2011). The right to health in the constitutions of member states of the World Health Organization South-East Asia Region. www.searo.who.int/entity/human_rights/documents/Health_and_Human_Rights_-_HHR_SEA-HHR-02.pdf?ua=1.

Wigley, S. and Akkoyunlu-Wigley, A. (2011). The impact of regime type on health: Does redistribution explain everything? *World Politics,* 63(4), 647–77.

Wildasin, D. (1997). *Fiscal Aspects of Evolving Federations*. Cambridge: Cambridge University Press.

Wildasin, D. E. (2008). Fiscal competition. In B. R. Weingast and D. A. Wittman (eds.). *The Oxford Handbook of Political Economy*. Oxford: Oxford University Press, pp. 502–20.

Wildavsky, A. (1987). Choosing preferences by constructing institutions: A cultural theory of preference formation. *American Political Science Review*, 81(1), 3–21.

Wilkinson, R. G. (1992). Income distribution and life expectancy. *BMJ: British Medical Journal*, 304(6820), 165.

Wilkinson, R. G. (1997). Socioeconomic determinants of health. Health inequalities: Relative or absolute material standards? *BMJ: British Medical Journal*, 314 (7080), 591.

Wirtz, V. J., Hogerzeil, H. V., Gray, A. L. et al. (2017). Essential medicines for universal health coverage. *The Lancet*, 389(10067), 403–76.

Wittman, D. (1973). Parties as utility maximizers. *American Political Science Review*, 67, 490–8.

Woodward, B., Drager, N., Beaglehole, R. and Lipson, D. (2002). Globalization, global public goods, and health. In N. Drager and C. Vieira (eds.), *Trade in Health Services: Global, Regional and Country Perspectives*. Washington, DC: Pan American Health Organization (PAHO), pp. 6–7.

Yin, W. (2008). Market incentives and pharmaceutical innovation. *Journal of Health Economics*, 27(4), 1060–77.

Zingales, L. (2017). Preventing economists' capture. In D. Carpenter and D. Moss (eds.), *Preventing Regulatory Capture: Special Interest Influence and How to Limit It*. New York: Cambridge University Press, pp. 124–51.

Zweifel, T. and Navia, P. (2000). Democracy, dictatorship and infant mortality. *Journal of Democracy*, 11, 99–114.

Index